Infection Prevention in the Perioperative Setting: Zero Tolerance for Infections

Guest Editor

GEORGE ALLEN, RN, PhD, MS, BSN, CIC, CNOR

PERIOPERATIVE NURSING CLINICS

www.periopnursing.theclinics.com

Consulting Editor
NANCY GIRARD, PhD, RN, FAAN

December 2010 • Volume 5 • Number 4

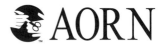

SAUNDERS an imprint of ELSEVIER, Inc.

W.B. SAUNDERS COMPANY

A Division of Elsevier Inc.

1600 John F. Kennedy Boulevard • Suite 1800 • Philadelphia, Pennsylvania 19103-2899

http://www.periopnursing.theclinics.com

PERIOPERATIVE NURSING CLINICS Volume 5, Number 4

December 2010 ISSN 1556-7931, ISBN-13: 978-1-4377-2482-0

Editor: Katie Hartner
Developmental Editor: Donald Mumford

Perioperative Nursing Clinics (ISSN 1556-7931) is published quarterly by Elsevier, 360 Park Avenue South, New York, NY 10010. Months of issue are March, June, September and December. Business and Editorial Offices: 1600 John F. Kennedy Blvd., Suite 1800, Philadelphia, PA 19103-2899. Customer Service Office: 11830 Westline Industrial Drive, St. Louis, MO 63146. Periodicals postage paid at New York, NY and at additional mailing offices. Subscription prices are $124.00 per year (domestic individuals), $213.00 per year (domestic institutions), $61.00.00 per year (domestic students/residents), $161.00 per year (international individuals), $245.00 per year (international institutions), and $65.00 per year (International students/residents). Foreign air speed delivery is included in all *Clinics* subscription prices. All prices are subject to change without notice. **POSTMASTER:** Send change of address to *Perioperative Nursing Clinics*, Customer Service (orders, claims, online, change of address): Elsevier Periodicals Customer Service, 11830 Westline Industrial Drive, St. Louis, MO 63146. Tel: 1-800-654-2452 (U.S. and Canada). Fax: 314-523-5170. E-mail: journals customerservice-usa@elsevier.com (for print support); journalsonlinesupport-usa@elsevier.com (for online support).

Reprints. For copies of 100 or more, of articles in this publication, please contact the Commercial Rights Department, Elsevier Inc., 360 Park Avenue South, New York, NY 10010-1710; Phone: (+1) 212-633-3813; Fax: (+1) 212-462-1935; E-mail: reprints@elsevier.com.

Printed in the United States of America.

Contributors

CONSULTING EDITOR

NANCY GIRARD, PhD, RN, FAAN
Nurse Collaborations, Boerne, Texas; Clinical Associate Professor, Acute Nursing Care
Department, University of Texas Health Science Center, San Antonio, Texas

GUEST EDITOR

GEORGE ALLEN, RN, PhD, MS, BSN, CIC, CNOR
Infection Preventionist, Director of Infection Control; Clinical Instructor, Department
of Epidemiology and Infection Control, State University of New York Downstate
Medical Center, Brooklyn, New York

AUTHORS

AUDREY B. ADAMS, RN, MPH, CIC
Director, Infection Prevention and Control Unit, Montefiore Medical Center, University
Hospital for the Albert Einstein College of Medicine, Bronx, New York

GEORGE ALLEN, RN, PhD, MS, BSN, CIC, CNOR
Infection Preventionist, Director of Infection Control; Clinical Instructor, Department
of Epidemiology and Infection Control, State University of New York Downstate
Medical Center, Brooklyn, New York

STEVEN BOCK, BA, BSN, RN, CIC
Infection Prevention and Control Specialist, Infection Prevention and Control Department,
New York University Langone Medical Center, New York, New York

ROBERT GARCIA, BS, MT (ASCP), CIC
Infection Preventionist, President and Founder, Enhanced Epidemiology, Valley Stream,
New York

LUCILLE H. HERRING, RN, BSN, MS, CIC
Infection Preventionist, Weiler Division, Montefiore Medical Center, Bronx, New York

MARY ANN MAGERL, RN, MA, CIC
Nurse Epidemiologist, Department of Infection Prevention and Control, Westchester
Medical Center, Valhalla, New York

KATHI MULLANEY, BSN, MPH, CIC
Senior Associate Director, Infection Control, Department of Infection Control, Metropolitan
Hospital, New York, New York

MARY OLIVERA, MS, CRCST, CHL, FCS
Clinical Specialist, Case Medical, Inc, South Hackensack, New Jersey

BARBARA A. SMITH, RN, BSN, MPA, CIC
Nurse Epidemiologist, Division of Infectious Diseases and Epidemiology, St Luke's
Roosevelt Hospital Center, New York, New York

Contents

Hand washing is the single most important procedure that health care personnel can perform before and after their interactions with patients to prevent the transmission of infections. In the perioperative setting, countless
skin-to-skin interactions requiring hand hygiene occur between health
care personnel and surgical patients. Noncompliance with recommended
hand hygiene requirements exposes patients to the development and/or
transmission of a wide range of infections, including multidrug-resistant
organism infections, surgical site infections, bloodstream infections, respiratory tract infections, and urinary tract infections. Infrastructural changes
and adopting a culture of safety can improve compliance to hand hygiene
recommendations and hence patient safety.

Multidrug-resistant organisms (MDROs) are recognized as a major public
health threat. Health care institutions are using various combined interventions for the prevention and control of MDROs. Such strategies include
improvements in hand hygiene, enforcing compliance with standard
precautions when caring for all patients, using contact precautions for patients known to be colonized and/or infected with MDROs, implementing
judicious antimicrobial procedures, implementing active surveillance for
targeted MDROs, educating personnel, providing enhanced cleaning procedures, and implementing decolonization procedures as appropriate for
targeted MDROs. In the perioperative setting, the focus is on using standard
precautions for all patients or contact precautions for patients identified as
colonized or infected with MDROs along with environmental sanitation.

Anesthesia is delivered in a variety of modalities including general, regional, or local. Patients are most vulnerable when receiving anesthesia,
as they must depend on the anesthesia team to provide this care without
untoward effects. It is expected that patients will be protected from health
care acquired infections (HAIs) by appropriate use of infection prevention
measures. In addition, the anesthesia team may be at risk of HAIs because
of their intimate contact with the patient's blood and respiratory system.

Adequate adherence to infection prevention methods should reduce the risk of occupation exposure and infection to the anesthesia team members. Health care associated infections involving anesthesia have been transmitted from health care worker to patient, patient to patient, and patient to the anesthesia provider. This article further discusses the risks for HAIs apparent in intravascular cannulation, endotracheal intubation, and the development of surgical site infections, and examines occupational measures to prevent infections in the health care worker. Regardless of the health care setting or the level of provider, the standard of care for infection prevention and managerial oversight of this care should remain the same.

The literature contains numerous articles that investigate and evaluate various aspects of SHA, such as the ideal length of hand disinfection for the surgical scrub, comparison of various scrub agents, effect of the surgical scrub on SSIs, and transition from the traditional hand scrubbing to hand rubbing with alcohol solutions. This article reviews some of these reports and provides some reactions of the surgical team regarding current surgical antisepsis protocols.

The use of a urinary catheter in patients undergoing surgery can vary substantially depending on the surgeon performing the procedure and the culture of the institution. Perioperative team members have a critical role in reducing the likelihood that a urinary catheter–associated infection develops. When urinary catheters are inserted in the operating room, personnel must pay scrupulous attention to the aseptic technique and keep the drainage bag below the level of the bladder.

The latest scientific information advances the knowledge of both methodology and type of antiseptic that should be used in most surgeries performed in the United States. The information contained here provides credible evidence that medical institutions should strongly consider revisions to their protocols that address skin antisepsis for their surgical patients.

At the author's hospital, perioperative services perform approximately 7,000 surgical procedures annually with 10% of the cases each year delayed or cancelled because of missing, mislabeled, or defective central sterile services instruments. Delays have the potential to negatively impact patient safety and operating room efficiency. The author and colleagues implemented the lean process, where the target state focused on eliminating cancellations or delays of operating room cases due to missing, mislabeled, or defective central sterile supply instruments. The results showed that when applied to a health care organization, lean principles can have a dramatic effect on improving processes and outcomes, reducing cost and cycle times, and increasing patient and staff satisfaction.

One component of the sterilization process is the biologic testing of sterilizers. Increased reports of biologic failures during flash sterilization provided an opportunity for improvement. This article identifies the cause of the biologic failures seen during flash sterilization to reduce the risks of endemic and epidemic infections in patients and to standardize the sterilization process throughout the surgical services.

Sharps-associated injuries continue to occur in the perioperative environment. Managers and administrators should develop policies and procedures that create a culture of safety for both patients and personnel. The core strategy for preventing sharps injuries must encompass the universal implementation of the Occupational Safety and Health Administration's Bloodborne Pathogen Standard and the understanding that sharps safety devices, whenever they are available in the marketplace, should be quickly and effectively incorporated into the institution operating procedures.

FORTHCOMING ISSUES

March 2011
Foot and Ankle Surgery
Thomas Zgonis, DPM, FACFAS,
Guest Editor

June 2011
Robotics
John Zender, RN, BS, CNOR,
Guest Editor

RECENT ISSUES

September 2010
**Sterilization and Disinfection for the
Perioperative Nurse**
Terri Goodman, PhD, RN, CNOR,
Guest Editor

June 2010
Radiology
Kathleen A. Gross, MSN, RN-BC, CRN,
Guest Editor

March 2010
Surgical Instruments
Kathleen B. Gaberson, PhD, RN, CNOR,
CNE, ANEF, *Guest Editor*

THE CLINICS ARE NOW AVAILABLE ONLINE!

Access your subscription at:
www.theclinics.com

Foreword

Zero Tolerance: No Lenience for Lack of Infection Control

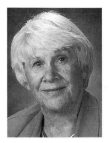

Nancy Girard, PhD, RN, FAAN
Consulting Editor

Ever since man was able to look through a microscope and see wee wiggling things, microorganisms have fascinated, infuriated, and frustrated us. This is as true today as it was in the distant past. The race to maintain, control, or eliminate life has been a major one for both humans and those pesky bugs. The battle has raged back and forth, at times with humans winning and at other times the microorganisms. However hard it is for us to admit, they have the ability to evolve and change to their environment faster and more effectively than we do and thus stay a step ahead. Microorganisms are becoming more virulent and resistant to antibiotics and other drugs developed to inhibit or stop their growth. As mankind develops new drugs, the microbes develop tolerance or structural changes. At the same time, drug companies are developing fewer new drugs to fight these microbes.

Today a crisis exists in the war against infections. The annual cost of treating infections in the U.S. is approximately $120 billion dollars. There are approximately 2 million health care associated infections (HAIs) that occur annually in the United States. It is further estimated that this leads to 60,000 to 90,000 deaths.[1] The most common infections are urinary tract infections, bloodstream infections, pneumonia, and surgical site infections.

All of the above factors have led to the next generation of warfare against controlling infection, moving from thresholds to zero tolerance. It is the hope that zero tolerance will lead to minimized or prevented infections with appropriate care. In addition to the moral and ethical need to prevent infections in the operating room, the pay-for-performance mandates from the Centers for Medicare and Medicaid Services provide further stimulus to prevent postoperative surgical infections.

It has become clear that the goal of zero tolerance cannot be accomplished by only one group of people (such as nurses) or by using only one procedure, such as

Perioperative Nursing Clinics 5 (2010) ix–xi
doi:10.1016/j.cpen.2010.09.005

handwashing (as important as it is). Infection control practitioners, as well as perioperative nurses, have long mandated proper infection control procedures. As good as they are, they are not enough. To win this battle (or at least control it as much as possible), every single person in the hospital must be involved, from administrators to those who clean the environment. There must be a culture strongly supported by all for zero tolerance for transmission of infections in the perioperative setting.

What does zero tolerance mean? It doesn't mean that there will never be another infection in the perioperative setting. It does mean that the transmission of infection-causing microbes by contact or air in the perioperative setting can and should be controlled. This is done by using infection prevention principles and best practices that are shown to be effective in minimizing transfer by contact or air. The operative setting is better at controlling spread of infection than most areas in the hospital, but hasn't stopped surgical wound infections. Having standards and policies are no good unless they are scrupulously followed by everyone. Zero tolerance means that sloppy techniques, ignorance of the procedures, or lack of policies cannot be allowed.[2] There has to be behavior modification and enforcement of best practices, as well as support from the highest administrator within the institution. Unfortunately, in many US hospitals, infection control programs are not well supported by administrators because they are not revenue-generating departments.

William Jarvis, MD, infection prevention expert, states that zero tolerance is "a culture, a goal, an attitude and a commitment. It uses effective tools such as evidence-based interventions in the form of bundles."[2] The worth of bundling care practices is being borne out by practitioners who are conducting research and quality improvement projects. It is becoming clear that bundled care processes are the most effective. These are practices that include all factors that can impact potential for infections. For example, these can include (but are not limited to) developing a culture for zero tolerance with a multidisciplinary team, enforcing and monitoring infection prevention in surgical areas and the operating room, monitoring and enforcing environmental cleaning and disinfection procedures for instruments. These, along with studies to investigate new technologies for reducing surgical site infections and resistant microorganisms, must be employed.[3]

Zero tolerance sounds good on paper. It is one of those concepts though, where operationalizing it takes tremendous effort from all involved. Murphy[4] provides the following 10-point plan for getting to zero:

1. Educate all health care providers about infection prevention
2. Educate hospital administration about infection prevention
3. Challenge health care workers to lead the charge against HAIs
4. Influence and educate stakeholders
5. Educate the community about infection prevention
6. Use and share meaningful infection data
7. Automate more tasks in infection prevention so more time is spent on education efforts
8. Learn how to make the business case for infection prevention
9. Develop strategic partnerships
10. Keep the patient at the center of all infection prevention efforts.

Zero tolerance means treating every infection as if it should never happen. However, in reality, some infections may still happen. When it does, we investigate the root cause. It means holding everyone accountable for HAIs. This is not a problem just for the infection control practitioners.

Managers in the perioperative setting should implement a zero tolerance for transmission of infections in the perioperative setting. Procedures are clearly defined that enforce aseptic techniques for insertion of urinary catheters, full barrier precautions and aseptic techniques for any invasive procedure, and strongly enforce compliance with hand hygiene recommendations, by all. Zero management teams should also develop and implement rational policies and procedures to identify and manage patients with multi-drug-resistant pathogens.

George Allen, the Guest Editor of this issue of *Perioperative Nursing Clinics*, noted, "Once we understand how important working as a team is, the more efficient we become, and the less likelihood we have of instances occurring. Like I said, two sets of eyes are always better than one—you can save a life by noticing something someone else didn't notice."[5]

Nancy Girard, PhD, RN, FAAN
Nurse Collaborations
8910 Buckskin Drive
Boerne, TX 78006-5565, USA

E-mail address:
Ngirard2@satx.rr.com

REFERENCES

1. Microbes/transmission. National Institution of Allergy and Infectious Disease. July 15, 2008. Available at: http://www.niaid.nih.gov/topics/microbes/understanding/transmission/pages/default.aspx. Accessed September 12, 2010.
2. Zero Tolerance for Infections. A Winning Strategy. Infection Control Today. January 24, 2008. Available at: http://www.infectioncontroltoday.com/articles/2008/01/zero-tolerance-for-infections-a-winning-strategy.aspx. Accessed September 12, 2010.
3. Spencer M. Working Toward Zero Surgical Site Infection Rate. Boston (MA), September 22, 2009. Podium presentation. ASHES Annual Conference. Reno (NV), September 20–24, 2009. Available at: http://www.ashes.org/ashes/conference/2009/content/ppt/spencer-maureen.pdf. Accessed September 12, 2010.
4. Murphy DM. Go for zero then pay it forward. APIC News. Fall 2007.
5. George Allen. AORN Q&A. Management Connection. October 2009. Available at: http://www.aorn.org/News/Managers/October2009Issue/ManagersQA. Accessed September 12, 2010.

Preface

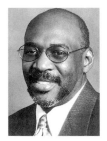

George Allen, RN, PhD,
MS, BSN, CIC, CNOR
Guest Editor

It is estimated that 50,000 deaths occur annually in hospitals in the United States among patients who have undergone surgical procedures.[1] A new report from the Centers for Disease Control and Prevention updates previous estimates of health-care-associated infections (HAI) reporting that HAI account for an estimated 1.7 million infections and 99,000 associated deaths each year. Of these infections, 32% of all HAI are urinary tract infections (UTI); 22% are surgical site infections (SSI); 15% are pneumonia (lung infections); and 14% are bloodstream infections (BSI).[2] Many believe that most of these perioperative adverse events are preventable, and that hospitals can improve operative outcomes through compliance with evidence-based procedures.[3] Indeed, the development of HAI, whatever the category we place them in—SSI, lung infection, BSI, or UTI—all can occur in patients undergoing surgical procedures and are preventable in most cases by the compliance with evidence-based practices, utilization of principles and concepts of continuous quality improvement, and embracement of a culture throughout the organization of zero tolerance for infection.

Unfortunately, the members of the surgical team are also at risk for the transmission of infections and must be included when adopting a culture of zero tolerance for infections in the perioperative setting. Principally their risk for getting an infection is by virtue of the extreme likelihood of having contact with the blood and other potentially infectious body fluids of patients undergoing surgical procedures. The Occupational Safety and Health Administration (OSHA) Bloodborne Exposure Standard provides evidence-based procedures—work practice controls and engineering controls, to reduce these exposures including requirements for health care facilities to institute procedures and protocols to prevent sharps exposures and offer hepatitis B vaccination free to all personnel who have potential risk of exposure to blood and body fluids of patients.[4] Additionally, perioperative personnel are also at risk for infections with multi-drug-resistant pathogens (MDROs) such as methicillin-resistant *Staphylococcus aureus*, *S aureus* with resistance to vancomycin, vancomycin-resistant enterococci, extended-spectrum

Perioperative Nursing Clinics 5 (2010) xiii–xv
doi:10.1016/j.cpen.2010.09.004
1556-7931/10/$ – see front matter © 2010 Elsevier Inc. All rights reserved.

periopnursing.theclinics.com

β-lactamase producing gram-negative bacilli, and *Clostridium difficile*, due to contact with patients who may potentially have these resistant bacteria. Here again, evidence-based recommendations are available to interrupt and prevent the transmission of MDROs, including isolation procedures, hand hygiene, and environmental cleaning protocols.[5-7]

Historically in the perioperative environment the emphasis has been on preventing the transmission and development of SSI. Consequently, there is wide compliance with evidence-based practices for preventing SSI, including those aimed at patients—preoperative showering with an antimicrobial agent; only removing hair from the operative site when it will interfere with the incision and only using clippers or a depilatory when hair removal is necessary; preparation of the incision site with an antimicrobial agent; timely administration of preoperative antibiotic prophylaxis; maintaining normothermia throughout the procedure; and controlling blood glucose levels. For the perioperative team members, compliance with hand hygiene recommendations for all contact with the patient; maintaining surgical asepsis; and being attuned to environmental sanitation and ventilation requirements are a must. However, the surgical team must understand that other types of infections can and do occur and institutionalize a culture of zero tolerance for all types of infection utilizing evidence-based practices. Evidence-based practices must be utilized each time a urinary catheter is inserted, each time a patient is intubated, and each time the vascular system is entered for the placement of peripheral or central venous access.

This issue is intended to emphasize the critical importance of compliance with basic infection control practices—utilizing evidence-based practices in concert with a culture of zero tolerance for infection specific to the perioperative experience for both health care personnel and patients. Articles in this issue include discussions on strategies for preventing injuries from sharp instruments and devices, discussion on managing patients with MDROs, discussion on the use of urinary catheters, information about how specific members of the surgical team such as the anesthesia care provider can positively impact patient safety and be a vital part of implementing a culture of zero tolerance for the transmission of infections, surgical skin preparation, hand hygiene, surgical hand antisepsis, maximizing procedures for instrument processing and availability, and using concepts and procedures from continuous performance improvements to drive change and improvements.

George Allen, RN, PhD, MS, BSN, CIC, CNOR
Department of Hospital Epidemiology and Infection Control
State University of New York
Downstate Medical Center
450 Clarkson Avenue, Box 1887
Brooklyn, NY 11203, USA

E-mail address:
George.allen@downstate.edu

REFERENCES

1. Merrill CT, Elixhauser A. Procedures in U.S. hospitals, 2003. HCUP Fact Book no. 7. Rockville (MD): Agency for Healthcare Research and Quality; 2006. Available at: http://www.ahrq.gov/data/hcup/factbk7/factbk7.pdf. AGRQ Publication No. 06-0039. Accessed September 14, 2010.

2. Centers for Disease Prevention and Control. Estimates of Healthcare-Associated Infections. Available at: http://www.cdc.gov/ncidod/dhqp/hai.html. Accessed September 14, 2010.
3. Brooke BS, Meguid RA, Makary MA, et al. Improving surgical outcomes through adoption of evidence-based process measures: intervention specific or associated with overall hospital quality? Surgery 2009;147(4):481–90.
4. U.S. Department of Labor. Occupational Safety and Health Administration, Bloodborne Pathogens Standard. Fed Regist 1991;56:64003–182 (29CFR 1910.1030).
5. Siegel JD, Rhinehart E, Jackson M, et al. Healthcare Infection Control Practices Advisory Committee. Guideline for isolation precautions: preventing transmission of infectious agents in healthcare settings. 2007. Available at: http://www.cdc.gov/ncidod/dhqp/pdf/isolation2007.pdf. Accessed September 14, 2010.
6. Boyce JM, Pittet D. Guidelines for hand hygiene in health-care settings: recommendations of the Healthcare Infection Control Advisory Committee and the HIPAC/SHEA/APIC/IDSA Hand Hygiene Task Force. MMWR Morb Mortal Wkly Rep 2002;51:1–45.
7. Recommended practices for environmental cleaning in the perioperative setting. Perioperative standards and recommended practices. Denver (CO): AORN Inc; 2010. p. 241–55.

Hand Hygiene and the Surgical Team

George Allen, RN, PhD, MS, BSN, CIC, CNOR

KEYWORDS

- Hand hygiene • Alcohol-based sanitizers
- Perioperative setting • Health care–associated infections

Health care–associated infections (HAIs) are a major cause of morbidity and mortality in health care institutions in the United States and throughout the world. These infections are associated with all aspects of health care delivery, from ambulatory care procedures to hospital admission and from general wards to intensive care units and long-term care facilities. HAIs are also associated with procedures performed in the perioperative setting from insertion of invasive devices and minimally invasive diagnostic and treatment modalities to surgical intervention and follow-up care and treatment. Such infections include urinary tract infections (UTIs), surgical site infections (SSIs), pneumonia (lung infections), and bloodstream infections. A recent report from the Centers for Disease Control and Prevention estimated the annual medical costs of treating HAIs in US hospitals to be between $28 billion and $45 billion, adjusted to 2007 dollars.[1] The potential for the transmission of multidrug-resistant organisms (MDROs), including methicillin-resistant *Staphylococcus aureus*; vancomycin-resistant strains of *Enterococci*; certain gram-negative bacteria, including those producing extended-spectrum β-lactamases; and *Clostridium difficile*, that are associated with higher morbidity and mortality, higher cost of treatment, and longer lengths of hospital stay than infections caused by other drug-sensitive organisms is increasing because these MDROs are becoming more and more prevalent in health care institutions and the society.[2]

HAIs account for an estimated 1.7 million infections and 99,000 associated deaths each year, with 32% UTIs, 22% SSIs, 15% pneumonia, and 14% bloodstream infections.[3] Hand hygiene, simply washing the hands with soap and water or using an alcohol-based waterless product if the hands are not visibly soiled, is universally thought to be the single most important procedure health care personnel can perform to prevent the transmission of HAIs.[4] However, the observed compliance rate in health care facilities has been regarded as unacceptably poor by public health authorities.[5] A recent review of compliance with hand hygiene in health care facilities concluded that noncompliance with hand hygiene guidelines is a universal problem; the overall

There are no financial disclosures.
Department of Epidemiology and Infection Control, SUNY Downstate Medical Center, 450 Clarkson Avenue, Box 1187, Brooklyn, NY 11203, USA
E-mail address: George.allen@downstate.edu

Perioperative Nursing Clinics 5 (2010) 411–418
doi:10.1016/j.cpen.2010.09.002
1556-7931/10/$ – see front matter © 2010 Elsevier Inc. All rights reserved.

median compliance rate was 40%, with unadjusted compliance rates lower in intensive care units (30%–40%) than in other settings (50%–60%), among physicians (32%) than among nurses (48%), and before (21%) contact with patients than after (47%).[6] Compliance with hand hygiene is a crucial step in preventing HAIs.

MITIGATING THE RISK OF INFECTION

Contamination of the surgical site with microorganisms is a necessary precursor for the development of an SSI, and the risk of an SSI has been conceptualized as the dose of the bacterial contamination multiplied by the virulence of the pathogens divided by the resistance of the host. In the development of SSIs, the source of pathogens is generally the endogenous flora of the patient's skin, mucous membranes, or hollow viscera. However, seeding of the operative site from a distant focus of infection and exogenous sources, including hands of members of the surgical team; the operating room environment; and equipments, tools, and instruments brought to the sterile field during the operation, also contribute to SSIs.[7]

UTIs are the most common type of HAI because of instrumentation of the urinary tract, necessitating the use of antimicrobials. The concomitant use of urinary drainage systems often provides the reservoir for multidrug-resistant bacteria and a source of transmission to other patients. The sources of microorganisms causing UTIs can be endogenous, via meatal, rectal, or vaginal colonization, or exogenous, such as on the hands of health care personnel or equipment. Indeed, pathogens enter the urinary tract either by the extraluminal route, migrating along the outside of the urinary catheter, or by the intraluminal route, moving along the internal lumen of the catheter from a contaminated collection bag or catheter drainage tube junction.[8] However, the hands of health care workers in the perioperative setting, including those of the anesthesia care provider during monitoring of bladder output or the circulating nurse positioning or securing the urinary catheter, tubing, or drainage bag, are a significant source of pathogens causing UTI.

Most health care–associated bloodstream infections stem from the use of central vascular catheters. Compared with peripheral venous catheters, which are frequently used in the perioperative setting, central vascular catheters carry a substantially greater risk for infection. Consequently, the level of barrier precautions needed to prevent bloodstream infection during central catheter insertion should be more stringent. Maximal barrier precautions, such as cap, mask, sterile gown, sterile gloves, and large sterile drapes, should be used during the insertion of the central catheter compared with only the use of standard precautions (sterile gloves and small drapes) for the insertion of a peripheral venous catheter. Migration of skin organisms at the insertion site into the cutaneous catheter tract along with colonization of the catheter tip is the most common route of infection for peripherally inserted catheters, resulting in bloodstream infections. Good hand hygiene before catheter insertion or maintenance combined with proper aseptic technique during catheter manipulation protects from bloodstream infection.[9]

High morbidity and mortality are associated with health care–associated pneumonia. Consequently, all semicritical items used in the respiratory tract during the administration of anesthesia in the perioperative setting, including face mask or tracheal tube, inspiratory and expiratory tubing, Y-piece and reservoir bag, humidifier, breathing circuits, fiberoptic bronchoscope, endotracheal tube, laryngoscope blade, mouthpiece, nebulizers and reservoirs, oral and nasal airways, resuscitation bags, stylets, and suction catheters, should be cleaned and disinfected or sterilized before use. Sterile water should be used for rinsing reusable semicritical items that have been subjected to a high level of chemical disinfection before use. Hands of health care workers must be decontaminated after contact with mucous membranes, respiratory secretions, or objects contaminated with respiratory secretions, regardless of wearing gloves, by washing with soap and water or using a waterless alcohol-based product if the hands are not visibly soiled. In addition, hands must be decontaminated before and after contact with a patient who has an endotracheal or a tracheotomy tube in place or with any respiratory device that is used on the patient.[10] However, there are numerous challenges in the perioperative milieu that must be overcome to facilitate an improvement in the hand hygiene compliance rates.

SURGICAL HAND SCRUB

Hand hygiene for the surgical team, perioperative nurses, surgeons, anesthesia care providers, surgical technicians and technologists, scrub personnel, transporters, and other unlicensed assistive personnel is inherently similar to what is required outside the perioperative setting in the other patient care areas. Hand hygiene is also an essential component of surgical hand scrub. The objective of the surgical hand scrub is to reduce the transient and resident flora on the hands of personnel (surgeons, scrub persons, and surgical assistants) who perform or assist in the surgical procedure. **Table 1** reviews the current recommended practices for the surgical hand scrub.[11]

HAND HYGIENE FOR THE SURGICAL TEAM

Hand hygiene for the surgical team requires that the hands be washed before and after every patient contact, before gloves are donned and after removal of the gloves, whenever hands are visibly soiled, and after touching contaminated surfaces or equipment. Effective hand hygiene involves washing the hand with soap and water for a minimum of 15 seconds using friction and paying attention to between the fingers and under the fingernails. A waterless alcohol-based hand rub product may also be used if hands are not visibly soiled or contact with spore-forming pathogens, including *C difficile*, is not suspected. **Box 1** outlines some of the major recommendations and steps for hand hygiene in the perioperative setting.[11] The World Health Organization has listed the following indications for hand hygiene:

1. Wash hands with soap and water when hands are visibly dirty or soiled with blood or other body fluids or after using the toilet.
2. If exposure to potential spore-forming pathogens is strongly suspected or proved, including outbreaks of *C difficile*, hand washing with soap and water is the preferred means.
3. Use an alcohol-based hand rub as the preferred means for routine hand antisepsis in all other clinical situations if hands are not visibly soiled. If an alcohol-based hand rub is not obtainable, wash hands with soap and water.
4. Perform hand hygiene before and after having direct contact with patients.
5. Perform hand hygiene before handling an invasive device for patient care regardless of the use of gloves.
6. Perform hand hygiene if moving from a contaminated body site to another body site during care of the same patient.
7. Perform hand hygiene after contact with inanimate surfaces and objects (including medical equipment) in the immediate vicinity of the patient.
8. Perform hand hygiene after removing sterile or nonsterile gloves.[12]

   Table 2 lists some of the common procedures that are followed in the perioperative setting that would require hand hygiene and the potential consequences of noncompliance. Managers in the perioperative setting must understand and effectively

Table 1 Surgical hand scrub	
Standardized Surgical Hand Scrub Using an Alcohol-Based Surgical Hand Rub Product	**Traditional Standardized Surgical Hand Scrub**
1. Remove jewelry, including rings, watches, and bracelets	1. Remove jewelry, including rings, watches, and bracelets
2. Don a surgical mask	2. Don a surgical mask
3. If hands are visibly soiled, prewash hands and forearms with plain soap and water or an antimicrobial agent	3. If hands are visibly soiled, prewash hands and forearms with plain soap and water or an antimicrobial agent
4. Clean the subungual areas of both hands under running water using a disposable nail cleaner	4. Clean the subungual areas of both hands under running water using a disposable nail cleaner
5. Rinse hands and forearms under running water	5. Rinse hands and forearms under running water
6. Dry hands and forearms thoroughly with a disposable paper towel	6. Dispense the approved antimicrobial scrub agent according to the manufacturer's written directions
7. Dispense the manufacturer-recommended amount of the surgical hand rub product	7. Apply the antimicrobial agent to wet hands and forearms using a soft nonabrasive sponge
8. Apply the product to the hands and forearms according to the manufacturer's written instructions	8. A 3- or 5-min scrub should be timed to allow adequate product contact with skin according to the manufacturer's written instructions
9. Repeat the product application as directed	9. Visualize each finger, hand, and arm as having 4 sides. Wash all four sides effectively, keeping the hands elevated. Repeat this process for the next hand, arm, and fingers
10. Rub thoroughly until completely dry	10. Avoid splashing surgical attire
11. Proceed to the operating room or other invasive procedure room and don a sterile surgical gown and gloves	11. Discard sponges, if used, in appropriate containers
	12. Rinse hands and arms under running water in one direction from the fingertips to the elbow as often as needed
	13. Hold hands higher than the elbows and away from the surgical attire
	14. In the operating room, dry hands and arms with a sterile towel before donning a sterile gown and gloves

communicate to the perioperative staff about the potentially serious consequence of a low level of compliance with hand hygiene, including the devastating consequences of SSI, pneumonia, bloodstream infection, and the potential for transmitting MDROs after developing a UTI.

TACKLING CHALLENGES TO COMPLIANCE WITH HAND HYGIENE IN THE PERIOPERATIVE SETTING

Addressing the challenges to achieving consistently high levels of compliance with hand hygiene in the perioperative setting begins with a commitment from the executive

Box 1
Recommendations for hand hygiene in the perioperative setting

The purpose of hand washing is to remove soil, organic material, and transient microorganisms from the fingernails, hands, and forearms to decrease the resident microorganism count to a minimum and to inhibit the rapid rebound of microorganisms.

Hand washing should be performed

Upon arrival at the health care facility

Before and after every patient contact

Before putting on gloves and after removing gloves or touching other personal protective equipment

Any time there is the possibility that there has been contact with blood or other potentially infectious materials or surfaces

Before and after eating

Before and after using the restroom

Before leaving the health care facility

When hands are visibly soiled

Table 2
Potential impact of noncompliance to hand hygiene requirements during the perioperative period

Patient Contact Requiring Hand Hygiene	Employee Type	Potential Consequences Because of Noncompliance
Preoperative		
Physical examination in the holding area	Surgeon/nurse/anesthesia provider	MDRO infection at any site
Assessing the airway	Anesthesia provider	Pneumonia
Marking the site	Surgeon	MDRO infection at any site
Inserting intravenous line	Anesthesia provider/nurse	Bloodstream infection/SSI
Inserting urinary catheter	Nurse	UTI/SSI
Administering oral medications	Nurse	MDRO infection at any site
Removal of hair	Nurse/surgeon	MDRO infection at any site
Transfer/positioning	Nurse/surgeon/UAP	MDRO infection at any site
Intraoperative		
Assessing intravenous site	Anesthesia provider/nurse	Bloodstream infection/SSI
Intubating	Anesthesia provider	Pneumonia/SSI
Oral suctioning	Anesthesia provider	Pneumonia
Counting used sponges	Nurse	MDRO infection at any site
Handling specimen	Nurse	MDRO infection at any site
Postoperative		
Transfer/moving	Nurse/UAP/anesthesia provider/surgeon	MDRO infection at any site/SSI
Assessing urinary catheter	Surgeon	
Assessing intravenous site	Anesthesia provider/nurse	Bloodstream infection/SSI
Assessing dressing site	Nurse	UTI/SSI

Abbreviation: UAP, unlicensed assistive personnel.

level of the institution's perioperative service to create and support a culture of safety and accountability. This culture of safety should include an ongoing assessment and evaluation of compliance with hand hygiene that is incorporated into the institution-wide hand hygiene program. The process for this assessment could be either direct observation or tabulation of the amount of hand hygiene products used over a period. Observational data on all levels of personnel should routinely be collected because they interact with patients daily. The data should be tabulated, aggregated, and reported back to the rank and file. In addition, the data should be used to provide and develop corrective actions when the rates are poor. Such actions include providing additional education as is indicated, developing and implementing additional hand hygiene reminder signage and posters, or adding infrastructure as is deemed necessary.[13]

Another challenge to compliance with hand hygiene in the perioperative setting is the accessibility to hand washing sinks. Hand washing sinks are not allowed in the room where surgery is being performed. However, there are numerous times during the intraoperative phase of the surgical procedures when hand hygiene is required. In many of those instances, it would be inappropriate for the health care worker to leave the room to perform hand hygiene. For the circulating room nurse, these instances include before donning gloves before inserting the urinary catheter or performing the surgical preparation; before and after assisting with positioning the patient, counting used sponges, and handling specimens; and after removing gloves. For the anesthesia care providers, these instances include before donning gloves for invasive procedures, such as the insertion of intravascular lines, performing spinal or block anesthesia techniques, oral suctioning of the patient, and/or touching the patient's mucous membranes, and after removal of gloves. For the surgeon, the surgeon's assistant, and the scrub personnel, these instances include after removal of personal protective equipments, including gloves, gowns, and goggles, and after a needlestick injury or cut. Perioperative managers and administrators should ensure that waterless alcohol-based hand hygiene products are readily available in the rooms where procedures are being performed. However, it is crucial that they be in compliance with the national and local fire codes. Because alcohol can support combustion, such hand hygiene dispensers should not be located over or next to sources of ignition, including electrical outlets and switches, lasers, or electrosurgical equipments.[13]

Preventing or reducing the potential for the transmission of MDROs in the perioperative setting is challenging because it is critically dependent on compliance with hand hygiene recommendations. MDROs are microorganisms that are resistant to commonly used antimicrobial agents. Patients colonized or infected with MDROs require special preparation and precautions. The most common route of transmission of MDROs is by contact with a contaminated person or object; thus, to prevent transmission, excellent hand hygiene practices, use of barriers, and careful cleaning of the environment must be done. Implementing isolation procedures with an emphasis on compliance with hand hygiene and environmental sanitation is an effective strategy. Consequently, facilities for hand hygiene must be readily available in each operating room.[14]

SUMMARY

Performing hand hygiene before and after every patient contact even when gloves are being used is the single most important procedure that all health care disciplines can perform to prevent the development and transmission of all types of infections. In the perioperative setting, such infections include bloodstream infections, pneumonia, UTIs, SSIs, and MDRO infections at all body sites. However, there are many challenges that perioperative administrators face to sustain high levels of compliance with the recommendations for hand hygiene. Such challenges include a requirement that hand washing sinks are not to be placed in the operating room, forcing personnel to leave the room to comply with hand hygiene requirements. Infrastructural changes, including the wide use of alcohol-based waterless hand hygiene products, and an administrative philosophy of commitment to evidence-based practices requiring monitoring and feedback of hand hygiene compliance rates can improve the safety of patients and staff in the perioperative setting.

REFERENCES

1. Scott RD. The direct medical costs of healthcare-associated infections in U.S. hospitals and the benefits of prevention. 2009. Available at: http://www.cdc.gov/ncidod/dhqp/pdf/Scott_CostPaper.pdf. Accessed August 15, 2010.
2. Siegel JD, Rhinehart E, Jackson M, The Healthcare Infection Control Practices Advisory Committee. 2007 Guideline for isolation precautions: preventing transmission of infectious agents in healthcare settings. 2007. Available at: http://www.cdc.gov/ncidod/dhqp/pdf/guidelines/Isolation2007.pdf. Accessed October 12, 2010.
3. Klevens RM, Edwards JR, Horan TC, et al. Estimating health care-associated infections and deaths in U.S. hospitals, 2002. Public Health Rep 2007;122:160–6.
4. Boyce JM, Pittet D. Guidelines for hand hygiene in health-care settings: recommendations of the Healthcare Infection Control Practices Advisory Committee and the HIPAC/SHEA/APIC/ISDA Hand Hygiene Task Force. MMWR Morb Mortal Wkly Rep 2005;51:1–45.
5. Day M. Chief medical officer names hand hygiene and organ donation as public health priorities. BMJ 2007;335(7611):113.
6. Erasmus V, Daha TJ, Richardus JH, et al. Systematic review of studies on compliance with hand hygiene guidelines in hospital care. Infect Control Hosp Epidemiol 2010;31(3):283–94.
7. Mangram AJ, Horan TC, Pearson ML, et al. Guideline for prevention of surgical site infection, 1999. Infect Control Hosp Epidemiol 1999;20(4):247–80. Available at: http://www.cdc.gov/ncidod/dhqp/pdf/guidelines/SSI.pdf. Accessed August 17, 2010.
8. Gould CV, Umscheid CA, Agarwal RK, et al. Guideline for prevention of catheter-associated urinary tract infections 2009. Atlanta (GA): Centers for Disease Control and Prevention. Healthcare Infection Control Practices Advisory Committee. Available at: http://www.cdc.gov/hicpac/pdf/CAUTI/CAUTIguideline2009final.pdf. Accessed August 17, 2010.
9. O'Grady NP, Alexander M, Dellinger EP, et al. Guidelines for the prevention of intravascular catheter-related infections. MMWR Recomm Rep 2002;51(RR10):1–26. Available at: http://www.cdc.gov/mmwr/preview/mmwrhtml/rr5110a1.htm. Accessed August 17, 2010.
10. Tablan OC, Anderson LJ, Besser R, et al. Guidelines for preventing health-care-associated pneumonia, 2003. MMWR Recomm Rep 2004;53(RR03):1–36. Available at: http://www.cdc.gov/mmwr/preview/mmwrhtml/rr5303a1.htm. Accessed August 17, 2010.
11. AORN. Recommended practices for hand hygiene in the perioperative setting. In: Retzlaff K, editor. Perioperative standards and recommended practices. Denver (CO): AORN, Inc; 2010. p. 75–89.

12. WHO. WHO guidelines on hand hygiene in health care: first global patient safety challenge. Clean care is safer care. Part II. Consensus recommendations. p. 152. Available at: http://whqlibdoc.who.int/publications/2009/9789241597906_eng.pdf. Accessed August 16, 2010.
13. Allen G. Hand hygiene: a patient safety issue in the perioperative environment. Perioper Nurs Clin 2008;3(2):101–6.
14. Williams TN, Haas JP. Multidrug-resistant pathogens: implementing contact isolation in the operating room. Perioper Nurs Clin 2008;3(2):149–53.

Managing Patients with Multidrug-Resistant Organisms: Implementing Isolation Precaution Procedures in the Perioperative Setting

George Allen, RN, PhD, MS, BSN, CIC, CNOR

KEYWORDS

- Multidrug-resistant pathogens • Colonization • Infection
- Isolation precautions • Prevention
- Environmental contamination • Transmission

Multidrug-resistant organisms (MDROs) are in general defined as microorganisms, predominantly bacteria, that are resistant to 1 or more classes of antimicrobial agents.[1] They usually are resistant to all but 1 or 2 commercially available antimicrobial agents.[2] The emergence of MDROs is increasingly recognized as a major public health threat. MDROs of clinical importance, which can be encountered in the perioperative setting (**Table 1**), include (1) methicillin-resistant *Staphylococcus aureus* (MRSA), (2) *S aureus* with resistance to vancomycin (vancomycin-intermediate *S aureus* [VISA]/vancomycin-resistant *S aureus* [VRSA]), (3) vancomycin-resistant enterococci (VRE), (4) extended-spectrum β-lactamases (ESBL)-producing gram-negative bacilli, and (5) *Clostridium difficile*. The escalating prevalence of MDROs during the last 2 decades poses several problems:

- Patients admitted to the hospital or scheduled for surgery may not have infections caused by MDROs. However, they may be known or not known to be colonized with MDROs and can thus transmit MDROs to other patients and health care personnel.
- Patients and residents from long-term care facilities with infections caused by MDROs are more likely to require hospitalization and may need surgical care,

There are no financial disclosures.
Department of Hospital Epidemiology & Infection Control, State University of New York (S.U.N.Y), Downstate Medical Center, 450 Clarkson Avenue Box 1887, Brooklyn, NY 11203, USA
E-mail address: George.allen@downstate.edu

Perioperative Nursing Clinics 5 (2010) 419–426
doi:10.1016/j.cpen.2010.07.003
1556-7931/10/$ – see front matter © 2010 Elsevier Inc. All rights reserved.

Table 1
Examples of clinically relevant MDROs

Agent	Reservoir	Mode of Transmission	Comments
MRSA	Colonized and infected patients Colonized HCWs Environment and fomites	Person-to-person HCW's hands Environment	Infections most often present as skin infections and is a major cause of surgical site infection Now endemic in most US hospitals MRSA-colonized patients are more likely to develop symptomatic infection than those with methicillin-sensitive *Staphylococcus aureus*
VISA VRSA	Colonized and infected patients Colonized HCWs Environment and fomites (24)	Person-to-person HCW's hands Environment	VISA and VRSA are rare in the United States Prolonged vancomycin use is a risk factor
VRE	GI, GU, and environment	Person-to-person HCW's hands Environment	Often multiresistant to penicillins and aminoglycosides
ESBL-producing GNB	GI	Person-to-person HCW's hands Environment	Resistant to cephalosporins and monobactam. Important ESBL-producing GNB include *Klebsiella pneumoniae, Pseudomonas aeruginosa, Serratia marcescens, Escherichia coli*

Resistant to multiple classes of antimicrobial agents	GI, GU, and environment	Person-to-person HCW's hands Environment	Strains of *Acinetobacter baumannii* resistant to all antimicrobial agents except imipenem (β-lactam antibiotic)
Organisms that are intrinsically resistant to the broadest-spectrum antimicrobial agents	GI, GU, and environment	Person-to-person HCW's hands Environment	*Stenotrophomonas maltophilia*, *Burkholderia cepacia*, and *Ralstonia pickettii*
Penicillin-resistant *Streptococcus pneumoniae*	Respiratory	Person-to-person Droplets Contact Saliva, coughing, fecal/oral	Resistant to penicillin and other broad-spectrum agents such as macrolides and fluoroquinolones
Clostridium difficile	Stool	Direct contact Environment Person-to-person HCW's hands	History of recent antimicrobial usage and diarrhea

Abbreviations: ESBL, extended-spectrum β-lactamase; GI, gastrointestinal; GNB, gram-negative bacilli; GU, genito urinary; HCW, health care worker; MRSA, methicillin-resistant *Staphylococcus aureus*; VISA, vancomycin-intermediate *S aureus*; VRE, vancomycin-resistant enterococci; VRSA, vancomycin-resistant *S aureus*.

resultingin increased costs and lengths of stay and adversely affected prognoses.[3–8]
- MDROs can spread to other patients and health care workers.
- The potential transfer of the genes transfers the resistance to other microorganisms.

Although *Klebsiella pneumoniae* carbapenemase (KPC)-producing *K pneumoniae* has emerged as an important health care–associated pathogen worldwide, the spread of its resistant plasmids into *Escherichia coli* is believed to pose an even greater public health risk, because resistant *E coli* may become part of the normal gut flora and thereby become a notable source of infection among sick and healthy persons in a health care setting. Such a transfer has occurred in 2008 when a carbapenem-non-susceptible *E coli* producing KPC-3 was isolated.[9]

TRANSMISSION OF MDROS

Once MDROs are introduced into a health care setting, transmission and persistence of these resistant strains are determined by several factors: the number and presence of susceptible or vulnerable patients, the pressure exerted by antimicrobial usage, the increased potential for transmission from larger numbers of patients who may be colonized or infected and have not been identified as carriers, and the effect of implementation and adherence to prevention efforts.

Colonization refers to the fact that the organism is present on or in the body but is not causing an infection, whereas infection means that the MDRO is present and causing illness. During the last several decades, the prevalence of MDROs in health care facilities in the United States has increased steadily with MRSA now accounting for more than 50% of the *S aureus* isolates. Similarly, the prevalence of VRE has increased from 1% to 15%, with VRE accounting for more than 28% of the enterococcus isolates. ESBL have also increased in prevalence with *Klebsiella* at 21% and *Pseudomonas* at 29%.[2] Gastrointestinal surgery and other types of gastrointestinal manipulations have been associated with *C difficile* infection, and the *C difficile* spores, which are resistant to most cleaning products, can remain in the environment for extended periods resulting in the potential for transmission to other patients and staff.[8]

Rapid detection of *S aureus* carriage followed by decolonization of the nasal and extranasal sites with mupirocin nasal ointment and bathing with chlorhexidine soap has been shown to be effective in reducing the risk for hospital-acquired infection with *S aureus*. It also reduced the mean length of hospital stay for patients suspected of being colonized or infected with MRSA.[10] Because of the morbidity and mortality associated with MDROs and the knowledge that patients colonized with MRSA are more likely to develop an infection, including surgical site infection, with MRSA than patients who are only colonized with methicillin-sensitive strains of *S aureus*,[6] identification of patients with MDROs is a critical step in reducing the likelihood of its transmission to other patients and staff. Current recommendations for preventing the transmission of MDROs in health care settings consist of the following:

Administrative measures and adherence monitoring
    Making MDRO prevention and control a patient-safety priority for the institution
    Providing the necessary administrative, human, and fiscal resources
    Implementing a multidisciplinary committee to improve adherence to recommended infection-control practices.

Education
> Providing training programs on all aspects of MDROs for all levels of health care workers.

Judicious use of antimicrobials
> Implementing a multidisciplinary committee to review antimicrobial use, resistance patterns, and the formulary
> Implementing a system to prompt clinicians to optimize the use of antimicrobial agents for specific isolates
> Providing clinicians with antimicrobial susceptibility reports and analysis, at least annually.

Surveillance
> Accurate identification of target MDROs
> Prompt notification to clinicians
> Monitoring trends over time
> Establishing a baseline for targeted MDROs
> Considering decolonization for targeted MDROs.

Infection control precautions
> Standard precautions
> Assessing indications for contact precautions.

Environmental measures
> Routine cleaning
> Isolation room cleaning.[2]

These recommendations must be tailored to specific locations within the institution. Consequently, personnel in the perioperative setting must develop and implement policies and procedures to reduce the likelihood of the transmission of MDROs to patients and persons during surgical procedures. The 2 areas of MDROs control germane to the perioperative setting are infection control and environmental measures.

INFECTION CONTROL MEASURES

Infection control measures to prevent the transmission of MDROs in patients scheduled for surgical procedures encompass 2 processes: the use of standard precautions or contact precautions for patients identified with MDROs along with a focus on environmental sanitation and cleaning of patient care equipments. Managers in the perioperative setting should develop and enforce written protocols for the process that they have decided is the most feasible based on their population, the prevalence of MDROs in their community and their institution, and their ability to identify patients colonized and/or infected with MDROs.

Standard Precautions

Standard precautions are intended to reduce the risk of transmission of blood-borne and other pathogens including MDROs from both recognized and unrecognized sources. Because colonization with MDROs is frequently undetected, standard precautions have an essential role in preventing transmission of MDROs in patients undergoing surgical procedures. The underlining principles of standard precautions are to consistently use prudent infection-prevention procedures such as hand hygiene and environmental cleaning for all patients, notwithstanding age, sex, type of surgery, length of the surgical procedure, or diagnosis of the patient. One of the recommended practices of the Association of periOperative Registered Nurses (AORN) is that health care workers should use standard precautions when caring for all patients in the perioperative setting.[11]

Hand hygiene is universally known as the single most important procedure to prevent the transmission of infections.[12] Hand hygiene is an important component of standard precautions. According to the standard precautions, hands must be washed before and after every patient contact, after touching patient care items, and whenever they are visibly soiled. Specific tasks commonly done in the perioperative environment require hand hygiene in addition to the situations mentioned earlier: performing a physical examination in the holding area, collecting specimens for laboratory examination, physical and visual inspection of the airway, removing hairs from the operative site, marking the operative site, administering nasal or face mask oxygen and medication (orally or by any other route), transferring the patient to the operating table, and positioning the patient for the surgical incision.

Hand hygiene involves the use of soap and water to vigorously rub the hands together for at least 15 seconds and then rinsing and drying. An alternative method is the use of the waterless alcohol-based product, which can be used if hands are not visibly soiled. The waterless alcohol-based product should not be used if the hands have visible soilage or when the patient is suspected or confirmed to have a spore forming pathogen, such as C difficile. Managers in the perioperative setting should provide hand washing facilities to facilitate compliance with hand hygiene in all areas of the perioperative environment where contact with patients is likely including the holding area where patients are interviewed and prepared for surgery, in the operating room where the patient is transferred to the operating table, and in the postanesthesia care unit (PACU) where the patients are cared for before being discharged or returned to their room. Because sinks cannot be placed within operating rooms, it is critical that hand hygiene stations (wall mounted dispensers, portable tabletop dispensers, foot pump–operated containers, or automatic dispensers) containing the alcohol-based waterless products be placed in strategic locations within each operating room where surgical and/or invasive procedures are being performed.[13]

Standard precautions include that in addition to compliance with hand hygiene, personnel must also routinely assess the risk of exposure to body fluids or contaminated surfaces and select and use personal protective equipment, such as gloves, fluid-resistant gowns, and/or face (mucous membrane) protective devices including masks with face shields or goggles when exposure is anticipated. Standard precautions also involve the use of respiratory hygiene and cough etiquette (covering the nose and mouth when coughing and sneezing) and environmental cleaning by using adequate procedures to routinely clean and disinfect environmental surfaces, equipment, and other frequently touched surfaces.

Contact Precautions

Contact precautions are intended to prevent transmission of infectious agents, including epidemiologically important microorganisms, such as MDROs, that are transmitted by direct or indirect contact with the patient or the patient's environment. AORN-recommended practices note that contact precautions should be used when care is being provided to patients who are known or suspected to be infected or colonized with microorganisms (including MDROs) that are transmitted by direct or indirect contact with patients or items and surfaces in the patient care environment.[11] To implement contact precautions in the perioperative setting, it is assumed that the patient is known to be colonized or infected with an MDRO. This information of the patient's health status must be communicated to the perioperative team at the time the procedure is booked to ensure that the applicable procedures are implemented before the patient is transferred to the operating room. Such patients should be transported directly to the operating room setup for the planned surgical procedure bypassing the holding area. The room should contain all the supplies and equipment needed for the planned surgical procedure. All unnecessary equipment and supplies should be removed from the room. The perioperative personnel caring for patients on contact precautions should wear a gown and gloves for all interactions that may involve contact with the patient or potentially contaminated areas in the patient's environment. Donning the gown and gloves on entry into the operating room and discarding them before exiting the operating room must be done to contain pathogens, especially those that have been implicated in transmission through environmental contamination, such as VRE, MRSA, and *C difficile*. Compliance with the hand hygiene recommendations discussed earlier is an essential component of contact precautions. After the surgical procedure, the need for continuing contact precautions must be communicated as a component of the transfer of care process to the staff in the PACU. Terminal cleaning as outlined in the AORN-recommended practice should be completed before another procedure is performed in the room. Terminal cleaning includes cleaning surgical lights and external tracts, fixed and ceiling mounted equipment, all furniture in the room including wheels and casters, handles of cabinets and push plates, ventilation faceplates and horizontal surfaces, the entire floor, kick buckets and scrub sinks.[14] It is important to understand that when *C difficile* is the MDRO, the cleaning solution should be a sodium hypochlorite product, because *C difficile* spores are resistant to the most commonly used environmental cleaning products.

SUMMARY

Preventing the transmission and spread of MDROs in health care settings is a national priority. Recommendations for preventing the emergence and transmission of these organisms require a comprehensive approach that includes administrative involvement and measures; education and training of health care personnel; judicious use of antimicrobial agents; comprehensive surveillance for targeted MDROs; application of infection control precautions such as standard precautions or contact precautions during patient care, environmental sanitation, cleaning and disinfection of the patient care environment and patient care equipment; and decolonization therapy when appropriate. In the perioperative setting during surgical procedures, preventing the transmission of MDROs can be accomplished by implementing and enforcing policies such as the use of standard precautions for all patients or the use of contact precautions for patients identified to be colonized or infected with MDROs. Compliance with hand hygiene is a core concept that is critical to any control process implemented in the perioperative environment.

REFERENCES

1. IOM. Appendix C: Glossary and acronyms. In: Harrison PF, Lederberg J, editors. Antimicrobial resistancle: issues and options. Workshop report. Washington, DC: National Academy Press; 1998. p. 8–74.
2. Siegel JD, Rhinehart E, Jackson M, et al, Healthcare Infection Control Practices Advisory Committee. Guideline for isolation precautions: preventing transmission of infectious agents in healthcare settings. Available at: http://www.cdc.gov/hicpac/pdf/isolation/Isolation2007.pdf. Accessed August 13, 2010.

3. Awad SS, Palacio CH, Subramanian A, et al. Implementation of a methicillin-resistant Staphylococcus aureus (MRSA) prevention bundle results in decreased MRSA surgical site infections. Am J Surg 2009;198(5):607–10.

4. Yano K, Minoda Y, Sakawa A, et al. Positive nasal culture of methicillin-resistant Staphylococcus aureus (MRSA) is a risk factor for surgical site infection in orthopedics. Acta Orthop 2009;80(4). DOI: 10.3109/17453670903110675. Available at: http://informahealthcare.com/doi/abs/10.3109/17453670903110675. Accessed August 13, 2010.

5. Imahara SD, Friedrich JB. Community-acquired methicillin-resistant *Staphylococcus aureus* in surgically treated hand infections. J Hand Surg Am 2010;35: 97–103.

6. Bode LG, Kluytmans JA, Wertheim HF, et al. Preventing surgical-site infections in nasal carriers of *Staphylococcus aureus*. N Engl J Med 2010;362(1):9–17.

7. Anderson DJ, Kaye KS, Chen LF, et al. Clinical and financial outcomes due to methicillin resistant *Staphylococcus aureus* surgical site infection: a multi-center matched outcome study. PLoS One 2009;4(12):e8305.

8. Gerding DN, Johnson S, Peterson LR, et al. Shea Position Paper. Clostridium difficile-associated diarrhea and colitis. Infect Control Hosp Epidemiol 1995;16(8): 459–77.

9. Goren MG, Carmeli Y, Schwaber MJ, et al. Transfer of carbapenem-resistant plasmid from *Klebsiella pneumoniae* ST258 to *Escherichia coli* in patient. Emerg Infect Dis 2010;16(6):1014–7.

10. van Rijen M, Bonten M, Wenzel R, et al. Mupirocin ointment for preventing *Staphylococcus aureus* infections in nasal carriers. Cochrane Database Syst Rev 2008; 4:CD006216.

11. Association of preOperative Registered Nurses. Recommended practices for prevention of transmissible infections in the perioperative practice setting. In: Perioperative standards and recommended practices. Denver (CO): AORN Inc; 2010. p. 277–87.

12. Boyce JM, Pittet D. Guidelines for hand hygiene in health-care settings: recommendations of the Healthcare Infection Control Practices Advisory Committee and the HICPA/SHEA/APIC/IDSA Hand Hygiene Task Force. MMWR Morb Mortal Wkly Rep 2002;51:1–45.

13. Allen G. Hand hygiene, an essential process in the OR [guest editorial]. AORN J 2005;82(4):561–2.

14. Association of preOperative Registered Nurses. Recommended practices for environmental cleaning in the perioperative setting. In: Perioperative standards and recommended practices. Denver (CO): AORN Inc; 2010. p. 241–55.

Anesthesia as a Risk for Health Care Acquired Infections

Barbara A. Smith, RN, BSN, MPA, CIC

KEYWORDS

- Health care infections • Anesthesia • Transmission

Modern health care relies on the provision of safe, effective anesthesia to patients undergoing surgery or other invasive procedures. It is perhaps while patients are receiving anesthesia that they are most vulnerable, as they must depend on the anesthesia team to provide this care without untoward effects. One expectation is that the patient will be protected from health care acquired infections (HAIs) by appropriate use of infection prevention measures. In addition, the anesthesia team may be at risk of HAIs because of their intimate contact with the patient's blood and respiratory system. Similarly, adequate adherence to infection prevention methods should reduce the risk of occupational exposure and infection to the anesthesia team members.

Health care associated infections involving anesthesia have been transmitted from health care worker to patient, patient to patient, and patient to the anesthesia provider. A recent report describes the development of bacterial meningitis in 5 women after intrapartum spinal anesthesia in which the route of transmission was from the anesthesiologist to the patient.[1] There have been several reports of patients acquiring viral hepatitis from other patients because of breaches in administration of parenteral anesthesia agents.[2,3] Occupational infections have occurred both through the contact route,[4] as with herpetic whitlow, and the respiratory route, as during the severe acute respiratory syndrome (SARS) outbreak in Toronto, Canada.[5]

Anesthesia is delivered in a variety of modalities including general, regional, or local anesthesia. The anesthetist's role has increasingly expanded to include the administration of other medications such as for conscious sedation or pain-alleviating drugs. While the anesthesia team has traditionally served in the operating rooms of acute care hospitals, their role has greatly expanded to ambulatory care centers, diagnostic, treatment, and procedure areas, pain management practices, and critical care units. This development has created a challenge for adherence to the highest standard of care for the prevention of infection. Regardless of the health care setting or the level

There are no financial disclosures.
Division of Infectious Diseases and Epidemiology, St Luke's Roosevelt Hospital Center, 1111 Amsterdam Avenue, New York, NY 10025, USA
E-mail address: basmith@chpnet.org

Perioperative Nursing Clinics 5 (2010) 427–441
doi:10.1016/j.cpen.2010.07.005

of provider, the standard of care for infection prevention and managerial oversight of this care should remain the same.

The anesthesia team has direct and indirect responsibility for the prevention of infections, which may manifest most commonly as bloodstream infections, local injection site infections, abscesses, meningitis, respiratory tract infections, and surgical site infections (SSIs). Bacterial and viral infections may also be attributed to anesthetic care.

Because anesthesia care interrupts two of the body's significant defense mechanisms, there is the potential for risk of infection to the patient.

First, the body's intact skin functions as a barrier to pathogenic organisms. However, intravascular cannulation for conscious sedation disrupts the skin integrity and permits a local or systemic infection to occur. These risks also apply to central venous vascular catheters inserted by the anesthesiologist, whether in the operating room or as part of a critical care team. Insertion of a needle, cannula, or implantable device into the spinal column for anesthesia or analgesia disrupts the skin integrity and provides a direct portal of entry for organisms.

Second, surgery will often be performed with general anesthesia that involves the insertion of an endotracheal tube to maintain an open airway and permit artificial ventilation during the procedure. Although endotracheal intubation during surgery is generally a controlled safe procedure, this artificial airway predisposes the body to exposure to respiratory pathogens whether from the health care provider, the environment, or equipment. The same risk arises when intubation is performed during an emergency situation such as cardiopulmonary resuscitation. Measures to prevent this exposure, including the role of the environment and equipment, are discussed in this article.

Third, although not physically involved at the sterile operative field, the anesthesia team can have influence over the development of SSIs by their collaboration with the surgical team in achieving normothermia, glycemic control, and appropriate antibiotic prophylaxis for the patient.[6]

Finally, the author examines occupational measures to prevent infections in the health care worker.

INFECTIOUS RISKS ASSOCIATED WITH THE INTERRUPTION OF THE SKIN BARRIER VIA DEVICES THAT PENETRATE THE SPINAL COLUMN

Access to the spinal column is used to provide regional anesthesia, for example with epidural anesthesia, or to deliver medication such as analgesics or steroids. Other examples of procedures that enter the spinal column include diagnostic procedures such as lumbar puncture and myelography.

The overall risk of infection from these procedures appears to be low. Miller[7] cites a rate of less than 1 per 10,000 cases of serious infection (ie, meningitis or spinal abscess). He notes 2 factors that had a relation to infection: the duration of epidural anesthesia and the patient's medical conditions. In a review conducted through 2005, Schulz-Stübner and colleagues[8] noted rates of 3.7 to 7.2 spinal abscesses per 100,000 cases and 0.2 to 83 epidural abscesses per 100,000 procedures. Baer[9] lists 179 cases of postdural meningitis occurring after spinal or epidural anesthesia and other types of instrumentation. Spinal or epidural anesthesia accounted for 65% of the cases (**Table 1**).

Some investigators have argued that the true incidence is unknown because there is no uniform reporting mechanism in the United States. Nonetheless, Ruppen and colleagues[10] attempt to define the risk in obstetric epidural anesthesia and cite a rate of 1 deep epidural infection per 145,000 procedures; an admittedly low

Table 1 Procedures causing postdural meningitis	
Spinal	96
Epidural	21
Myelography	29
Diagnostic lumbar puncture	17
Combined spinal-epidural	10
Steroid injection	2

Data from Baer E. Post dural puncture meningitis. Anesthesiology 2006;105(2):381–93.

incidence. Nonetheless, in an American Society of Anesthesiology newsletter, Hughes[11] urges his obstetric colleagues that they can lower the risk to their patients.

Evidence of infection transmission is also documented in the descriptions of outbreaks. Five women in two separate states (New York and Ohio) developed bacterial meningitis after intrapartum anesthesia (**Table 2**).[1] The article reveals that the causative organism was recovered from a nasal swab of one of the anesthesiologists linked to the 2 cases in Ohio. In each outbreak, unmasked personnel (including the anesthesiologist delivering the spinal anesthesia in Ohio) were present in the room during the procedures.

Eight cases of meningitis following myelography were reported by the Centers for Disease Control and Prevention (CDC) that appear related to contamination from mouth flora from the clinicians who performed the procedure.[12] As part of the investigation, the CDC eliminated equipment and fluids as a potential source for these infections, and confirmed that adequate aseptic technique had been followed.

As described by Baer,[9] the mechanism of infection in these cases occurs through:

- Droplet transmission of aerosolized mouth organisms,
- Contamination from skin bacteria or
- Hematogenous or direct spread from an endogenous site of infection.

Regarding this first method of transmission, the likelihood is that some of these infections are related to the clinician who performed the procedure. This assumption is supported by arguments that several cases were related to clusters among specific operators, or were linked by DNA testing of nasal swabs from the operator and positive cerebrospinal fluid cultures, as in the Ohio case cited.

These data suggest that the clinician can implement preventive practices related to anesthesia or analgesia given through the spinal cord to reduce the likelihood of infection. These practices include skin disinfection with an appropriate antiseptic, sterile

Table 2 Description of cases of meningitis after spinal anesthesia			
Location	No. of Women	Organism	Outcome
New York	3	Streptococcus salivarius in 2 patients No growth in 1 patient	All recovered
Ohio	2	S salivarius both patients	One recovered One expired

Data from Centers for Disease Control and Prevention. Bacterial meningitis after intrapartum spinal anesthesia—New York and Ohio, 2008–2009. MMWR Morb Mortal Wkly Rep 2010;59:65–9.

gloves and sterile drapes, and aseptic technique. Because of the growing evidence for droplet transmission of oropharyngeal flora during the procedures that puncture the spinal column, the CDC's Guidelines for Isolation Precautions recommend the use of a surgical mask by personnel placing a catheter or injecting material into the spinal canal or subdural space.[12] A recent practice advisory prepared by the American Society of Anesthesiologists (ASA) concurs with the implementation of aseptic technique when handling neuraxial needles and catheters, and states it should include "hand washing, wearing of sterile gloves, wearing of caps, wearing of masks covering both the mouth and nose, use of individual packets of skin preparation, and sterile draping of the patient." The same advisory does not make a specific recommendation regarding the type of skin antisepsis to use.[13]

INFECTIOUS RISKS ASSOCIATED WITH THE INTERRUPTION OF THE SKIN BARRIER VIA DEVICES THAT ENTER THE INTRAVASCULAR SYSTEM

Intravascular catheters, including central and peripheral venous catheters and arterial catheters, play an integral part in the delivery of anesthesia or analgesia. Once again, these devices provide an opportunity for organisms to enter the normally sterile vasculature.

The insertion and care of these catheters should remain the same regardless of whether they are inserted in an operating room, a critical care unit or a free-standing practice.

There are 2 key mechanisms by which a catheter can lead to an infection.[14] The first occurs with colonization of the device and is referred to as catheter-associated infection. The pathogenesis of these types of infections is:

- Skin organisms gain entry via the puncture site at time of insertion or shortly thereafter,
- The catheter hub can become contaminated during use or
- Organisms spread hematogenously from another site of infection in the body.

Catheter-associated infections can lead to local site infections or systemic infections including bacteremia, sepsis, or endocarditis.

The second mechanism occurs with contamination of the medication or substance being injected, which is referred to as infusate-associated infection. Although intrinsic contamination of intravenous fluids or medications from the manufacturer is rare in the United States, improper procedures by the anesthetist or technician during medication preparation and administration can led to infusate-associated infections. In this situation the bacteria, virus, or fungus is directly infused into the patient's bloodstream.

CATHETER-ASSOCIATED AND INFUSATE-ASSOCIATED INFECTION

The rate of catheter-associated infections varies by the type of device used. For peripherally inserted, short-term catheters the risk is low. Lee and colleagues[15] report a local site infection rate of 2.1% to 2.6% among 3165 patients with short peripheral intravenous catheters. No patients in this group developed a bloodstream infection. Rates of arterial line catheter infections are similarly low, with Lucet and colleagues[16] and Koh and colleagues[17] reporting rates of 1.0 and 0.92 bacteremias per 1000 catheter days, respectively. These investigators report low rates of bacteremias related to central venous lines as well. The risk of central line–associated bloodstream infections in critical care patients ranges from 1.3 infections per 1000 catheter days in pediatric medical units to 5.5 in burn units.[18] **Table 3** lists the central line–associated bloodstream infection rates in a sample of units in which the anesthetist may have involvement.

Table 3 Central line–associated bloodstream infection rate per 1000 central venous line days in selected units	
Critical Care Units	
Neurosurgical	2.5
Pediatric cardiothoracic	3.3
Surgical	2.3
Surgical cardiothoracic	1.4
Trauma	3.6
Inpatient Wards	
Labor, delivery, postpartum	0.0
Neurosurgical	0.9
Orthopedic	0.8
Surgical	1.4

Data from Edwards JR, Peterson K, Mu Y, et al. National Healthcare Safety Network report (NHSN): data summary for 2006 through 2008, issued December 2009. Am J Infect Control 2009;37:783–805.

Although it is possible for individual solutions to become contaminated and subsequently infused into patients, it is difficult to attribute an individual infection to a specific medication, vial, or infusion bag without direct causal evidence. Hence, data related to infusate-related infections derives mainly from experiences with outbreaks. For example, Blossom and colleagues[19] describe an outbreak of 162 *Serratia marcescens* bacteremias in 9 states related to manufacturer's contamination of prefilled heparin and saline syringes. These circumstances are clearly beyond the control of the anesthesia team, although the team must respond promptly to alerts regarding potential contamination. There are, however, reports of medication contamination occurring under the control of the anesthesia personnel.

In 2003, *Morbidity and Mortality Weekly Report* reported hepatitis B and C virus transmission occurring in 3 separate locations.[3] In each of these practices, reuse of needles and syringes and contamination of multidose medication vials led to patient-to-patient transmission of viral infections. As depicted in **Table 4**, more than 200 people were affected.

Despite this significant number of patient-to-patient transmissions, practitioners have continued to demonstrate unsafe medication practice. As recently as 2008, 6 patients were infected with hepatitis C due to unsafe injection practice used during sedation for endoscopic procedures.[2] The investigation revealed that the anesthesia provider contaminated vials of propofol by repeated aspiration into the vial with a syringe contaminated with hepatitis C from backflow of the index patient's blood. Although the vial was labeled for single-patient use, the practitioner used the vial on the next patients. A graphical example is shown in **Fig. 1**.

MEASURES TO PREVENT CATHETER-ASSOCIATED AND INFUSATE-ASSOCIATED INFECTIONS

The CDC has published extensive guidelines for the prevention of intravascular infections.[20] Key elements intended to reduce catheter-associated infections that

Table 4
Summary of hepatitis B and C transmission in 3 outpatient settings

Location	Practice Setting	Improper Techniques	Patients Infected
New York City	Endoscopy practice	Contamination of MDV of anesthesia medication	12: hepatitis C
New York City	Medical office	Contamination of MDV used for IM injections	29: hepatitis B
Oklahoma	Pain management	Reuse of needle and syringe for sedatives	69: hepatitis C 31: hepatitis B
Nebraska	Hematology-oncology practice	Use of single IV flush bag during infusions to multiple patients	99: hepatitis C

Abbreviations: IM, intramuscular; IV, intravenous; MDV, multidose vial.

Data from Centers for Disease Control and Prevention. Transmission of hepatitis B and C viruses in outpatient settings: New York, Oklahoma and Nebraska, 2000–2002. MMWR Morb Mortal Wkly Rep 2003;52:901–6.

apply to peripheral, central, or arterial catheters handled by the anesthesia team include:

- Skin disinfection of the intravenous insertion site with an appropriate disinfection (a chlorhexidine-based preparation is preferred),
- Aseptic technique during insertion and care and
- Decontamination of ports and stopcocks with a disinfectant such as 70% alcohol before accessing the device.

The CDC guidelines and the ASA recommend additional specifications for the insertion and maintenance of central venous catheters because of their higher risk of infection.[21] Many facilities have adopted a bundle approach to the insertion of central line catheters both in the operating room and elsewhere. The elements of the bundle are:

1. Hand hygiene before insertion
2. Full barrier precautions: sterile gown, gloves, masks, and large sterile drapes
3. Skin antisepsis with chlorhexidine
4. Subclavian vein as preferred anatomic site versus internal jugular or femoral
5. Daily review of line necessity.

From the anesthetist's perspective, the elimination of infusate-related infections demands preventing contamination of medications and infusions. Most practitioners presumably would report adherence to safe medication handling. Yet a survey conducted by the American Association of Nurse Anesthetists (AANA) revealed that 1% to 3% of clinicians reuse needles or syringes on multiple patients.[22] The AANA has joined with the CDC, two state medical societies, the Association for Practitioners in Infection Control, and other advocacy groups in the Safe Injection Practices and Awareness Campaign to further educate health care providers and the public about the importance of these practices. The campaign poster is displayed in **Fig. 2.**[23]

Because of the aforementioned outbreaks of hepatitis transmission, the CDC's 2007 Guidelines for Isolation Precautions[12] highlights safe injection practices that

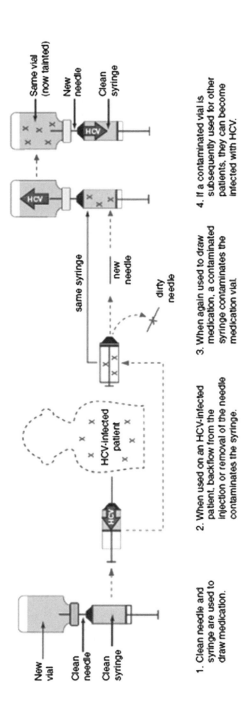
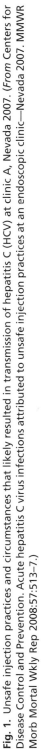

1. Clean needle and syringe are used to draw medication.

2. When used on an HCV-infected patient, backflow from the injection or removal of the needle contaminates the syringe.

3. When again used to draw medication, a contaminated syringe contaminates the medication vial.

4. If a contaminated vial is subsequently used for other patients, they can become infected with HCV.

Fig. 1. Unsafe injection practices and circumstances that likely resulted in transmission of hepatitis C (HCV) at clinic A, Nevada 2007. (*From* Centers for Disease Control and Prevention. Acute hepatitis C virus infections attributed to unsafe injection practices at an endoscopic clinic—Nevada 2007. MMWR Morb Mortal Wkly Rep 2008;57:513–7.)

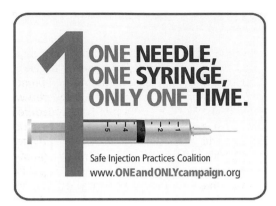

Fig. 2. Poster for safe injection practices. (*Courtesy of* S. Weir, Safe Injection Practices Coalition—One and Only Campaign; with permission.)

are outlined in **Fig. 3**. The ASA supports these practices[21] and makes further recommendations:

- Cleanse rubber septum of vials and the neck of glass ampoules with a disinfectant.
- Medications should be drawn up as close as possible to the time of use.
- Medications in a syringe should be discarded within 24 hours unless specified by the manufacturer or pharmacy.
- Expiration times for medications must be followed, especially the time limits for the use of lipid formulations such as propofol.

- Never administer medications from the same syringe to more than one patient, even if the needle is changed.
- Consider a syringe or needle contaminated after it has been used to enter or connect to a patients' intravenous infusion bag or administration set.
- Do not enter a vial with a used syringe or needle.
- Never use medications packaged as single-use vials for more than one patient.
- Assign medications packaged as multi-use vials to a single patient whenever possible.
- Do not use bags or bottles of intravenous solution as a common source of supply for more than one patient.
- Follow proper infection-control practices during the preparation and administration of injected medications.

Fig. 3. Injection safety recommendations. (*Adapted from* the Centers of Disease Control. Guideline for isolation precautions: preventing transmission of infectious agents in health-care setting 2007. Atlanta (GA): US Department of Health and Human Services, CDC; 2007. Available at: http://www.cdc.gov/ncidod/dhqp/gl_isolation.html.)

RISKS OF INFECTION RELATED TO INTUBATION, MECHANICAL VENTILATION, AND ANESTHESIA EQUIPMENT

According to the National Health Care Safety Network, the range of postprocedure pneumonias varies greatly by procedure.[18] For example, among those procedures reporting more than 1000 cases, patients undergoing knee prosthesis had a rate of 0.06 postoperative pneumonias per 100 procedures compared with cardiac surgery patients who had a rate of 1.19 pneumonias per 100 procedures. Some additional information is gleaned from examining rates of ventilator-associated pneumonias (VAP). Among surgical type critical care units, the pooled mean rate per 1000 ventilator days was a low of 0.6 in pediatric cardiothoracic units to a high of 8.1 in trauma units. However, it is difficult to distinguish how much of a direct impact intubation and anesthesia had on the development of these pneumonias. One study by Rello and colleagues[24] examined the development of pneumonia within the first 48 hours of intubation. Eighteen of 250 intensive care unit (ICU) patients developed pneumonia within the first 24 hours. There were 65 surgical patients included in this study. The 2 most important risk factors for pneumonia in patients were undergoing cardiopulmonary resuscitation and receiving conscious sedation. The investigators conclude that variables directly related to the intubation had less of an impact on the occurrence of pneumonia.

Nonetheless, intubation places the patient at risk of infection for several reasons. Because intubation interrupts the defense mechanisms of the upper airway, it increases the risk of aspiration. Aspiration of oral pharyngeal secretions is a prime cause of health care acquired pneumonia. This condition may be further aggravated by mechanical damage to the larynx or trachea from the endotracheal tube or stylet.[7] Furthermore, mechanical ventilation increases the risk of infection.

Measures to reduce infection risk associated with intubation and mechanical ventilation deal with technique and equipment. Cheung and colleagues[25] reviewed the literature to determine the impact of sterile handing of the endotracheal tube and the incidence of pneumonia. Of note, the investigators found very few data on the topic yet noted that intubations performed under unsterile conditions do occur, although they do not provide a recommendation. It is prudent for intubation to be performed as aseptically as possible, with personal protective equipment worn for the safety of the health care worker.

Oral intubation is preferred over nasal intubation because the latter is more likely to lead to sinusitis, thereby increasing the risk of aspiration of infected secretions.[26] Care should be taken to drain condensate in the ventilator tubing away from the patient. Although there are other measures to reduce VAP such as mouth care and semirecumbent position of the patient, these apply after the intraoperative period.

Equipment utilized by the anesthesia team includes endotracheal tubes, laryngoscope handles and blades, fiberoptic endoscopes, and anesthesia circuits, machines, and carts. There are also ancillary devices used by the team such as pulse oximetry, invasive temperature probes, and airways. This equipment may become contaminated from contact with the patient's skin, blood, secretions, splashes from the operative field, or contact with contaminated hands of the health care worker. The CDC, ASA, and AANA each have comparable standards for cleaning and disinfection of these items. These standards are based on the Spaulding classification method[27] that stratifies items based on their likely contact with a sterile body site, mucus membrane, or intact skin, as noted in **Table 5**.

Neither the CDC[12] nor the ASA[21] recommends the routine use of a bacterial filter for the breathing circuits or anesthesia ventilators. Conversely, the AANA states "protective

Table 5
Spaulding classification regarding disinfection and sterilization as applied to anesthesia equipment

Risk	Definition	Reprocessing Method	Examples
Critical items	Enter a sterile area of the body or vascular system	Require sterilization	Vascular needles Needles and catheters used for regional blocks
Semicritical items	Contact mucous membranes but do not penetrate them	High-level disinfection	Laryngoscope blades Esophageal catheters Stylets
Noncritical items	Touch intact skin or do not make contact with the patient	Intermediate- to low-level disinfection	Electrocardiogram cables Exterior of the anesthesia machine

From Centers for Disease Control and Prevention. Guideline for disinfection and sterilization in healthcare facilities, 2008. Available at: http://www.cdc.gov/hicpac/pdf/guidelines/Disinfection_Nov_2008.pdf.

use of bacterial filters is recommended," although they do acknowledge its use is controversial.[28] Each of these organizations supports the use of a bacterial filter when caring for an infectious tuberculosis patient. Another debated topic is the disinfection of laryngoscope handles. Because they do not enter sterile tissue or touch mucous membranes, the Spaulding classification would indicate cleaning and low-level disinfection. There is, however, the risk of contamination with body fluids. Call and colleagues[29] challenged a common practice of wiping blades with low-level disinfectant between operative cases. After culturing 40 handles that had been cleaned according to the facilities' standard practice, they found 75% had positive bacterial cultures.

Most importantly, standard protocols should be developed that outline the correct cleaning, disinfection, or sterilization process for each item used by the anesthesia team. The manufacturer of the equipment should be consulted for their recommendations. An oversight mechanism should be included in the policy to ensure adherence with the correct practice. Adequate training must be provided.

Overall, the documented transmission of infection from anesthesia equipment appears to be low. Yet Loftus and colleagues[30] raise the issue of transmission of bacteria in the anesthesia work area. These investigators cultured 2 specific areas of the anesthesia machine and the sterile stopcock just before the beginning of the case and again at the end of the case. Their results showed that 32% of the stopcocks were contaminated by the end of the case. The work area showed a significant increase in bacterial contamination as well. Two cases of methicillin-resistant *Staphylococcus aureus* (MRSA) were transmitted to the work area intraoperatively. One case of vancomycin-resistant *Enterococcus* transmission was documented between the anesthesia work are and the stopcock. The investigators also noted a trend toward increased HAIs among patients with contaminated stopcocks. The machine and stopcocks appear to have become contaminated by contact with providers' hands or lapses in aseptic technique.

These results reinforce the need for rigorous attention to hand hygiene not only before the start of surgery but also intraoperatively. Most studies indicate that adherence to hand hygiene by health care workers needs to be improved. McGuckin and colleagues[31] report only modest improvement to 51% compliance among non-ICU staff after a year-long program of observation and feedback. A 2004 report by Pittet and colleagues[32] found a 23% compliance rate among anesthesiologists. Hand hygiene is clearly a challenge in the operating room because of the multiple functions being performed. Limited access to hand hygiene products within the operating room undoubtedly contributes to poor compliance in the room.

Koff and colleagues[33] address this latter challenge through a study utilizing a portable device that dispenses alcohol-based hand rub. The device has the added benefit of tracking the frequency of use and providing a reminder if too long a time has elapsed between hand hygiene events. The introduction of the device was considered the study phase. During the study phase, hand hygiene events increased among attending anesthesiologists and other caregivers by 6.9 and 8.3 times per hour, respectively. The investigators also monitored the frequency of stopcock contamination and the occurrence of HAIs, and demonstrated decreases in both of these indicators as noted in **Table 6**. While the reduction in HAIs is promising, Koff and colleagues caution that additional research is needed to confirm these results.

ADDITIONAL ROLES FOR THE ANESTHESIA TEAM IN PREVENTION OF SURGICAL SITE INFECTIONS

SSIs are the second most frequent HAI.[34] Control measures for the prevention of SSIs include preoperative preparation of the patient, sterile attire and draping, surgical hand preparation, skin antisepsis, air handling, and sterile surgical instrumentation. There are additional conditions that can influence the occurrence of SSIs when the anesthesiologist may be involved.

One measure aimed at reducing bacteria at the surgical site is the delivery of antibiotic prophylaxis. The National Surgical Infection Prevention Project (SIP) proposes a 25% reduction in national surgical complication rates by adherence to 3 indicators[35]:

1. Administration of an appropriate antibiotic as described by the SIP. The antibiotic is selected based on the organisms most likely to cause infection and varies by the type of surgery.

Table 6
Results of use of portable hand hygiene device on stopcock contamination and HAIs

	Control Group	Study Group
Number of procedures	58	53
Stopcock contamination	32.8%	7.5%
HAIs	17.2%	3.8%
Types of HAIs	2 VAPs 5 wound 2 bloodstream 1 UTI	2 wound

Abbreviations: UTI, urinary tract infection; VAP, ventilator-associated pneumonia.
Data from Koff M, Loftus R, Burchman C, et al. Reduction in intraoperative bacterial contamination of peripheral intravenous tubing through the use of a novel device. Anesthesiology 2009; 110:978–85.

2. Timely administration of the antibiotic. To reach adequate blood and tissue concentrations, the antibiotic should be administered within the 60 minutes prior to the surgical incision. (Vancomycin may be given up to 120 minutes prior.)
3. Discontinuation of prophylactic antibiotics with 24 hours (48 hours for cardiac surgery).

A second intervention to reduce SSIs is the maintenance of normothermia. Hypothermia is thought to contribute to infection because of a decrease in subcutaneous tissue perfusion.[6] Lastly, glycemic control has been shown to reduce the rate of infections.

PREVENTION OF INFECTIONS IN ANESTHESIA PERSONNEL

Anesthesia providers are at risk of occupational infections from direct contact with blood and respiratory secretions. In addition, they may be exposed to microorganisms via the airborne or droplet route.

Diseases transmitted through the airborne route include tuberculosis, measles, and varicella. Most clinicians should be immune to measles and varicella because of effective vaccines. Surgery should be delayed for patients with these active infections. If the case cannot be postponed, the air handling in the operating room should ideally have negative pressure relative to the corridor. As previously mentioned, a bacterial filter should be placed on the anesthesia breathing circuit for patients with active tuberculosis. The health care provider should wear an N95 respirator approved by the National Institute for Occupational Safety and Health. When called to intubate patients on airborne isolation, again the N95 respirator is indicated. A large number of SARS cases in Canada were occupationally acquired. Fowler and colleagues[5] determined in one small series that physicians and nurses involved in intubation had a relative risk of 3.82 and 13.29, respectively, of developing SARS. This result stresses adequate respiratory protection.

Infections spread through the droplet route include pertussis, mumps, and influenza. As most of these cases are unlikely to undergo elective surgery or procedures while symptomatic, the exposure may occur from undiagnosed cases or from people who are shedding organisms in the few days prior to symptoms. Respiratory protection is indicated for known or suspect cases. Immunization is strongly encouraged. (For the 2009–2010 influenza season, the CDC recommended use of an N95 for contact with patients with influenza-like symptoms. Current recommendations can be found at http://www.cdc.gov/flu/professionals.) Hand hygiene in indicated.

Because of their contact with blood and other body fluids, anesthesia providers may be exposed to viral pathogens such as hepatitis B or C and human immunodeficiency virus (HIV). It is difficult to determine the actual number of occupationally acquired blood-borne infections in the discipline. In a 1998 study among anesthesia personnel, the estimated average 30-year risks of HIV or hepatitis C virus infection per full-time equivalent was 0.049% and 0.45%, respectively.[36]

In addition, there may be exposure to bacterial pathogens such as MRSA and *Clostridium difficile*. The AANA supports the CDC's recommendations to use standard precautions in the care of all patients.[28] In summary, standard precautions entail:

- Consider all blood and body fluid as potentially infectious.
- Use of personal protective equipment (PPE) (gloves, gowns, protective eye wear, and masks) when anticipating contact with blood or body. The PPE worn will depend on the task being performed and the possibility that splash or aerosolization can occur.
- Handle and dispose of all needles and syringes properly.

The practitioner should be aware of his or her facility's protocol for managing occupational exposure to blood and body fluid. Body fluid exposures should be evaluated promptly to determine the need for antiviral or other prophylaxis.

Transmission-based precautions may be added for particular diseases that are highly transmissible or of epidemiologic importance. There are 3 categories: airborne isolation, droplet precautions, and contact precautions.

SUMMARY

The documented risk of infection related to anesthesia is low, yet the potential exists for serious infectious outcomes including death. The risk of infection can be minimized by adherence to hand hygiene, aseptic technique, safe infection practices, equipment decontamination, and use of PPE by all members of the anesthesia team.

REFERENCES

1. Centers for Disease Control and Prevention. Bacterial meningitis after intrapartum spinal anesthesia—New York and Ohio, 2008–2009. MMWR Morb Mortal Wkly Rep 2010;59(3):65–9.
2. Centers for Disease Control and Prevention. Acute hepatitis C virus infections attributed to unsafe injection practices at an endoscopic clinic—Nevada 2007. MMWR Morb Mortal Wkly Rep 2008;57(19):513–7.
3. Centers for Disease Control and Prevention. Transmission of hepatitis B and C viruses in outpatient settings: New York, Oklahoma and Nebraska, 2000–2002. MMWR Morb Mortal Wkly Rep 2003;52(38):901–6.
4. Barash P, Cullen B, Stoelting R. Clinical anesthesia. Philadelphia: Lippincott, Williams and Wilkins; 2006. p. 85.
5. Fowler R, Guest C, Lapinsky S. Treatment of severe acute respiratory syndrome during intubation and mechanical ventilation. Am J Respir Crit Care Med 2004; 169(11):1198–202.
6. Mauermann W, Nemergut E. The anesthesiologist's role in the prevention of surgical sire infection. Anesthesiology 2006;105(2):413–21.
7. In: Miller RD, editor. Anesthesia. 6th edition. Philadelphia: Elsevier/Churchill Livingstone; 2005. p. 2742–3.
8. Schulz-Stübner S, Pottinger JM, Coffin SA, et al. Nosocomial infections and infection control in regional anesthesia. Acta Anaesthesiol Scand 2008;52(8):1144–57.
9. Baer E. Post dural puncture meningitis. Anesthesiology 2006;105(2):381–93.
10. Ruppen W, McQuay H, Moore R. Incidence of epidural hematoma, infection and neurologic injury in obstetric patients with epidural analgesia/anesthesia. Anesthesiology 2006;105(20):394–9.
11. Hughes S. Neuraxial blockade in obstetrics and complications related to infection: can we lower the risk? Park Ridge (IL): American Society of Anesthesiology newsletter. February, 2007;vol. 71. Available at: http://www.asahq.org/newsletters/2007/02-07/hugehs02_07.html. Accessed February 7, 2010.
12. Siegel J, Rhinehart E, Jackson M, et al, Centers for Disease Control and Prevention. Guideline for isolation precautions: preventing transmission of infectious agents in healthcare settings. 2007. Available at: http://www.cdc.gov/hicpac/2007IP/2007isolationPrecautions.html. Accessed January 20, 2010.
13. Horlocker T, Birnbach D, Connis R. Practice Advisory for the prevention, diagnosis, and management of infectious complications associated with neuraxial techniques: a report by the American Society of Anesthesiologists task force

on infectious complications associated with neuraxial techniques. Anesthesiology 2010;112(3):530–45.

14. Crnich C, Maki D. Intravascular device infection. In: Carrico R, editor. APIC text of infection control and epidemiology. 3rd edition. Washington, DC: APIC; 2009. p. 24:1–24:22.

15. Lee WC, Chen HL, Tsai T, et al. Risk factors for peripheral intravenous catheter infection in hospitalized patients: a prospective study of 3165 patients. Am J Infect Control 2009;37(8):683–6.

16. Lucet JC, Boudama L, Zahar JR. Infectious risk associated with arterial catheters compared to central venous catheters. Crit Care Med 2010;38:1030–5. Accessed February 26, 2010.

17. Koh DB, Gowardman JR, Rickard CM, et al. Prospective study of peripheral arterial catheter infection and comparison with concurrently sited central venous catheters. Crit Care Med 2008;36(2):397–402.

18. Edwards JR, Peterson K, Mu Y, et al. National healthcare safety network report (NHSN): data summary for 2006 through 2008, issued December 2009. Am J Infect Control 2009;37:783–805.

19. Blossom D, Nobel-Wang J, Su J. Multistate outbreak of *Serratia marcescens* bloodstream infections caused by contamination of prefilled heparin and isotonic sodium chloride solution syringes. Intern Med 2009;169(18): 1705–11.

20. Centers for Disease Control and Prevention. Guidelines for prevention of intravascular catheter-related infections. MMWR Morb Mortal Wkly Rep 2002;51 (RR10):1–26.

21. American Society of Anesthesiologists. Recommendations for infection control for the practice of anesthesiology. 2nd edition. Park Ridge (IL): ASA Publications; 1999.

22. American Association of Nurse Anesthetists. AANA condemns unsafe injection practice. Press release. March 6, 2008. Available at: http://www.aana.com/news.aspx?id=12396&terms=safe+injection. Accessed February 14, 2010.

23. One and Only Campaign. Available at: http://67.228.183.132/%7Ehardtime/OneandOnly/index.html. Accessed February 24, 2010.

24. Rello J, Diaz E, Roque M, et al. Risk factors for developing pneumonia within 48 hours of intubation. Am J Respir Crit Care Med 1999;159(6):1742–6.

25. Cheung N, Dotro G, Luckianow G et al. Endotracheal intubation: the role of sterility. Surg Infect (Larchmt) 2007;8(5):545–52.

26. Peyrani P. Pneumonia. In: Carrico R, editor. APIC text of infection control and epidemiology. 3rd edition. Washington, DC: APIC; 2009. p. 24:1–24:22.

27. Rutala W, Weber D, and the HICPAC, Centers for Disease Control and Prevention. Guideline for disinfection and sterilization in healthcare facilities, 2008. Available at: http://www.cdc.gov/hicpac/pdf/guidelines/Disinfection_Nov_2008.pdf. Accessed February 7, 2010.

28. American Association of Nurse Anesthetists. AANA Infection control guide for certified nurse anesthetists. Park Ridge (IL): AANA; 1997.

29. Call T, Auerbach F, Riddell S. Nosocomial contamination of laryngoscope handles: challenging current guidelines. Anesth Analg 2009;109(2):479–83.

30. Loftus R, Koff M, Burchman C, et al. transmission of pathogenic bacterial organisms in the anesthesia work area. Anesthesiology 2008;109:399–407.

31. McGuckin M, Waterman R, Govednik J. Hand hygiene compliance rates in the United States—a one year multicenter collaboration using product/volume usage measurement and feedback. Am J Med Qual 2009;24(3):205–13.

32. Pittet D, Simon A, Hugonnet S, et al. Hand hygiene among physicians: performance, beliefs and perceptions. Ann Intern Med 2004;141(1):1–8.
33. Koff M, Loftus R, Burchman C, et al. Reduction in intraoperative bacterial contamination of peripheral intravenous tubing through the use of a novel device. Anesthesiology 2009;110(5):978–85.
34. Fry D, Howard R. Surgical site infections. In: Carrico R, editor. APIC Text of infection control and epidemiology. 3rd edition. Washington, DC: APIC; 2009. p. 23:1–23:11.
35. QualityNet. Available at: http://www.qualitynet.org/dcs/ContentServer?c=MQParents&pagename=Medqic%2FContent%2FParentShellTemplate&cid=1228694349383&parentName=Category. Accessed March 1, 2010.
36. Greene E, Berry A, Jagger J, et al. Multicenter study of contaminated percutaneous injuries in anesthesia personnel. Anesthesiology 1998;89(6):1362.

Surgical Hand Antisepsis: Where We Have Been and Where We Are Today

Audrey B. Adams, RN, MPH, CIC

KEYWORDS

- Surgical hand antisepsis • Hand hygiene
- Surgical site infection • Hand scrub

The purpose of surgical hand antisepsis (SHA) is to prevent surgical site infections (SSIs) by reducing the transient and resident flora on the hands of operating team members while maintaining bacterial levels below baseline and thus reducing the likelihood of the introduction of organisms into the surgical wound.[1–3] SHA is the primary line of defense to remove transient flora, decrease the population of bacterial resident flora, and provide persistent antimicrobial activity. Gloves are the secondary line of defense to prevent transmission of organisms during surgical procedures. However, on average, 18.2% and 4.2% of undetected perforations have been found in the case of single and double gloving, respectively.[4] These potential leaks in gloves may allow both transient and resident hand flora to enter body cavities during surgery.

The literature contains numerous articles that investigate and evaluate various aspects of SHA, such as the ideal length of hand disinfection for the surgical scrub, comparison of various scrub agents, effect of the surgical scrub on SSIs, and transition from the traditional hand scrubbing to hand rubbing with alcohol solutions. This article reviews some of these reports and provides some reactions of the surgical team regarding current surgical antisepsis protocols.

WHERE WE HAVE BEEN

European countries have provided a great volume of literature on SHA.

It has been reported that although guidelines for standardized methods to evaluate antibacterial activity of antiseptics are available in several countries, the absence of an internationally agreed on test makes comparing study findings difficult.

In 1958, the German Society of Hygiene and Microbiology published the first standardized test method for the evaluation of surgical hand disinfection procedures.[5]

Infection Prevention and Control Unit, Montefiore Medical Center, University Hospital for the Albert Einstein College of Medicine, 111 East 210th Street, Bronx, NY 10467, USA
E-mail address: aadams@montefiore.org

Perioperative Nursing Clinics 5 (2010) 443–448
doi:10.1016/j.cpen.2010.07.001
1556-7931/10/$ – see front matter © 2010 Elsevier Inc. All rights reserved.

periopnursing.theclinics.com

Sixty percent n-propyl alcohol was established as the reference substance, with an application time of 5 minutes. Revised guidelines that were published in 1981 maintained the same requirements, and agents that met these requirements were listed as suitable for SHA with an exposure time of 5 minutes. Over time, other European countries published results showing a range of exposure times from 2 to 5 minutes.

In 1991, Babb and colleagues[6] published "A test procedure for evaluating surgical hand disinfection," which showed that after 2 minutes of 70% isopropanol application, suitable log reductions for immediate and sustained effects were achieved. Traditionally, surgical staff were required to scrub for 10 minutes, which frequently leads to skin damage. Several published studies demonstrated that a 5-minute scrub reduced bacterial counts as effectively as a 10-minute scrub. In addition, other studies demonstrated that bacterial counts reduced to acceptable levels were achieved after 2- or 3-minute surgical scrubbing.

In 1992, Hingst and colleagues[5] performed a comparative investigation of 7 basic substances and agents, which included a combination of different alcohols, quaternary ammonium compounds, povidone-iodine (PVP-I), and chlorhexidine. The tests were performed to investigate whether it was possible to reduce the application time to 3 minutes without losing efficiency in both the immediate and the prolonged effect of bacterial reduction. There were 6 serial experiments performed on 20 volunteers, all of whom had no visible skin lesions on their hands. Product A, 60% n-propyl alcohol, was used as the standard reference agent. The 3-minute application time could achieve the desired results for certain agents tested, depending on the formula and type of active substance. The investigators concluded that 60% n-propyl alcohol proved to still be the most effective preparation and that other preparations containing chlorhexidine were more effective with a higher percentage of alcohol base. Hingst and colleagues suggested that standard test procedures were needed to evaluate the essential need for sustained reduction value after 3 hours. The investigators also emphasized that a shorter period of 1 or 2 hours for the determination of sustained values may be more adequate for clinical purposes if surgeons perform a series of short operations, not exceeding 60 minutes in each case.

Aksoy and colleagues[7] investigated the factors that affect surgical hand disinfection with polyvidone iodine. Hands of 100 operating staff (75 doctors, 25 nurses) were tested before and after washing and after the surgical procedure by pressing the fingertips of both hands on agar culture. The investigators found that there was a significant decrease in the number of organisms on the hands when hand washing lasted longer than 3 minutes compared with hand washing that lasted less than 3 minutes; when surgery lasted longer than 95 minutes, the number of colonies was significantly higher. Aksoy and colleagues concluded that to attain effective disinfection with polyvidone iodine, SHA should be for at least 3 minutes. The recolonization risk increases when the duration of surgery exceeds 95 minutes.

In 1995, Paulson[8] published a comparative evaluation of surgical hand scrub preparations. The investigator stated that the literature contained articles that reported the antimicrobial effects of commonly used surgical products; however, none that directly compared the 3 parameters of efficacy or antimicrobial properties could be found:

1. Immediate (inactivation of organisms at the skin surface within 60 seconds of completing SHA)
2. Persistent (antimicrobial effectiveness lasting 6 hours postscrub)
3. Residual (cumulative antimicrobial properties after use for a period).

A study was designed to evaluate these 3 parameters in 5 surgical scrub products: 4% chlorhexidine (CHG), 2% CHG, PVP-I, parachlorometaxylenol (PCMX), and alcohol. The evaluation demonstrated that the 2 CHG products caused a significant immediate reduction in the organism count and demonstrated persistent and residual efficacy. The iodophor product had effective immediate and persistent properties but did not show significant residual effects. PCMX demonstrated low-level immediate and persistent effects but no residual antimicrobial effects. The investigator concluded that CHG products are the most favorable surgical hand scrub preparations.

WHERE WE ARE TODAY

The landmark 2002 Guideline for Hand Hygiene of the Healthcare Infection Control Practices Advisory Committee (HICPAC) and the HICPAC/Society of Healthcare Epidemiology of America (SHEA)/Association for Professionals in Infection Control and Epidemiology/Infectious Disease Society of America Hand Hygiene Task Force[9] provided an exhaustive review of the scientific data (423 references) regarding hand hygiene and revised standards of practice. The review of SHA acknowledged the numerous articles that demonstrated that using a brush or sponge was not necessary to reduce bacterial counts on hands during a surgical scrub, especially when alcohol-based products are used. Category 1B recommendations were made for 3 SHA recommendations. This 1B category indicates a strong recommendation for implementation, which is supported by certain experimental, clinical, or epidemiologic studies and a strong theoretical rationale. The three 1B SHA recommendations include the following:

1. Use an antimicrobial soap or an alcohol-based hand rub with persistent activity for SHA.
2. When using an antimicrobial soap, scrub hands and forearms for the length of time as recommended by the manufacturer, usually 2 to 6 minutes. Long scrub times (eg, 10 minutes) are not necessary.
3. Follow the manufacturer's instructions when using an alcohol-based surgical hand scrub product with persistent activity or prewash hands and forearms with a nonantimicrobial soap and dry hands and forearms completely before applying the alcohol solution.

This relaxed recommendation created a paradigm shift from the traditional approach of surgical hand scrub to surgical hand rub antisepsis. In 2005, the Centers for Disease Control and Prevention (CDC)/HICPAC guidelines were accepted as a standard of practice by the Association of periOperative Registered Nurses (AORN).[10] Current AORN guidelines recommend that SHA be performed by members of the surgical team (surgeon, assistants, and scrub nurse or surgical technician) before donning sterile gloves using either an antimicrobial surgical scrub agent intended for SHA or an alcohol-based antiseptic surgical hand rub with documented persistent and cumulative activity.[11] Hand-rubbing protocols are rapidly being offered as an alternative to hand scrubbing in many institutions. Evaluations of this paradigm shift are appearing in the literature.

Carro and colleagues[12] performed an in-use microbiological comparison of 2 surgical hand disinfection techniques in cardiothoracic surgery: hand rubbing versus hand scrubbing. Recognizing the role of presurgical hand disinfection on influencing the risk of SSIs, the investigators compared the microbial efficacy of the 2 techniques, using fingertip impressions before and immediately after disinfection, every 2 hours, and at the end of the operation. The surgical team alternately used the 2 techniques every 2 weeks from February to April 2003. Acceptability of hand rubbing was assessed by a questionnaire. Bacterial counts were comparable for both techniques immediately after hand disinfection, but the counts were significantly lower in the hand rub group at the end of surgery. Bacterial skin flora reduction immediately after hand disinfection, after 2 and 4 hours of operating time, and at the end of surgery was better in the hand rub group. The acceptability of hand rubbing was excellent, and the investigators concluded that the surgical hand rub disinfection was a valid alternative to the conventional hand-scrubbing protocol.

Parienti and colleagues[13] reported a randomized equivalence study on hand rubbing with an aqueous alcoholic solution versus traditional surgical hand scrubbing and 30-day SSI rates. The investigators concluded that the hand-rubbing solution preceded by a 1-minute nonantiseptic hand wash before each surgeon's first procedure of the day and before any other procedure if hands were soiled was as effective as the traditional hand scrub. There was no significant difference in the SSI rates between hand-scrubbing and hand-rubbing techniques. The surgical team had better tolerance of the hand-rubbing technique, and improved compliance with the hand hygiene guidelines was reported.

Berman[14] performed an evaluation in an acute care hospital in the southeastern United States to examine brushless scrubbing before laminectomy, craniotomy, and colectomy procedures. No increase in SSIs was identified when the brushless surgical product was used. A survey work sheet was completed to evaluate the overall satisfaction with the brushless product; there were a total of 324 data collection forms. More variation in response was noted when postoperative skin integrity was compared with the preoperative state. Nurses and surgical technicians reported worse skin conditions (problems maintaining skin moisture over time) than surgeons and house physicians after brushless scrubbing. This observation was attributed to the increased frequency of surgical scrubs by nurses and surgical technicians. No differences were noted among the staff regarding the time expenditure and ease of use variables. Overall, participants were pleased with the use of the brushless product.

An abstract titled "Knowledge, practice and opinions of surgical staff one year after implementing the use of an alcohol-based surgical hand scrub product" was presented during a SHEA conference poster session by the author in 2005.[15] A total of 109 survey responses from 53 surgeons (49%), 36 nurses (33%), 10 operating room (OR) technicians (9%), and 10 physician assistants (9%) were analyzed. There were 8 knowledge questions; 46% of the participants were not aware that chlorhexidine gluconate was a component of the product, and 91% did not select the correct duration of antimicrobial activity of the product. The average correct response to the 6 remaining knowledge questions was 87%. Practice questions disclosed that 30% of the respondents always preprepared hands and nails appropriately before using the product and 58% complied with spreading the remaining hand preparation over the hand and above the elbow. From the opinion questions, it was found that the product was preferred over traditional hand preparation by 42% of the respondents. Forty-six percent agreed that their hand condition had not improved. The data disclosed that among respondents who used the product, 47% continued to prefer the traditional scrub, whereas 42% preferred the new product. Knowledge and practice questions revealed a need for product in-service education during orientation and compliance monitoring. Only 46% thought that the product had improved hand conditions, suggesting the need for continued product development.

SUMMARY

The understanding of hand antisepsis has progressed over the years.

The enormous volume of published research on hand hygiene, reviewed by CDC/HICPAC, has provided the solid foundation for their hand hygiene recommendations. Performance indicators are included in the recommendation for measuring and monitoring compliance with hand hygiene and feedback to personnel.

Health care facilities should be encouraged to expand this effort of performance improvement to SHA in the OR setting. The CDC/HICPAC guidelines stated that although the studies reviewed were not designed to assess the independent contribution of hand hygiene on the prevention of hospital-acquired infections, the results demonstrated that improved hand hygiene practices reduced the risk of transmission of pathogenic organisms. Compliance with the established standards of SHA can contribute to improving quality and patient safety in the surgical arena.

REFERENCES

1. Centers for Disease Control and Prevention. Guideline for hand hygiene in health-care settings. MMWR Recomm Rep 2002;51(RR–16):1–44.
2. Widmer AE, Dangel M. Alcohol-based handrub: evaluation of technique and microbiological efficacy with international infection control professionals. Infect Control Hosp Epidemiol 2004;25(3):207–9.
3. Rotter ML, Kampf G, Suchomel M, et al. Long term effect of a 1.5 minute surgical hand rub with a propanol-based product on the resident hand flora. J Hosp Infect 2007;66(1):84–5.
4. Kraig N, Bei M, Hoffman, et al. [Surgical gloves-how well do they protect against infection?]. Gesundheitswesen 1999;61:398–403 [in German].
5. Hingst V, Juditzki I, Heeg P, et al. Evaluation of the efficacy of surgical hand disinfection following a reduced application time of 3 instead of 5 minutes. J Hosp Infect 1992;20:79–86.
6. Babb JR, Davies JG, Ayliffe GA. A test procedure for evaluating surgical hand disinfection. J Hosp Infect 1991;18(Suppl B):41–9.
7. Aksoy A, Caglayan F, Cakmak M, et al. An investigation of the factors that affect surgical hand disinfection with polyvidone iodine. J Hosp Infect 2005;16:15–9.
8. Paulson D. Comparative evaluation of five surgical hand scrub preparations. AORN J 1994;60:246–56.
9. Boyce JM, Pittet D, Healthcare Infection Control Practices Advisory Committee, HICPAC/SHEA/APIC/IDSA Hand Hygiene Task Force. Guideline for hand hygiene in health-care settings. Recommendations of the Healthcare Infection Control Practices Advisory Committee and the HICPAC/SHEA/APIC/IDSA Hand Hygiene Task Force. Society for Healthcare Epidemiology of America/Association for Professionals in Infection Control/Infectious Diseases Society of America. MMWR Recomm Rep 2002;51:1–45.
10. Recommended practices for surgical hand antisepsis/hand scrubs. In: Standards and recommended practices. Denver (CO): AORN, Inc; 2005. p. 377–85.
11. Recommended practices for hand hygiene in the perioperative setting. In: Perioperative standards and recommended practices. Denver (CO): AORN, Inc; 2010. p. 75–89.
12. Carro C, Camilleri L, Traore O, et al. An in-use microbiological comparison of two surgical hand disinfection techniques in cardiothoracic surgery: hand rubbing versus hand scrubbing. J Hosp Infect 2007;67:62–6.

13. Parienti J, Thibon P, Heller R, et al. Hand-rubbing with an aqueous alcoholic solution versus traditional surgical hand-scrubbing and 30-day surgical site infection rates. JAMA 2002;288:722–7.
14. Berman M. One hospital's clinical evaluation of brushless scrubbing. AORN J 2004;79:349–58.
15. Adams A, Bevan M, Herring L, et al. Knowledge, practice and opinions of surgical staff one year after implementing the use of an alcohol-based surgical hand-scrub product [abstract]. APIC Conference. Baltimore (MD) June 19–23, 2005.

Catheter-Associated Urinary Tract Infection Prevention in Surgical Patients

Steven Bock, BA, BSN, RN, CIC

KEYWORDS

- Urinary catheters • Intraluminal contamination
- Extraluminal contamination

Urinary catheters are among the most commonly used indwelling medical devices in hospitalized patients. The first modern indwelling urinary catheter was invented by a urological surgeon, Frederic Foley, in 1929. Refinements to the device led to the design that was patented in the 1930s. The modern Foley catheter is virtually the same as the originally designed device, except for the materials from which it is made.[1]

Because an indwelling urinary catheter serves as a continuous conduit from the bladder to the outside of the body and functions, in the reverse, as a means for external microorganisms to gain access to the bladder, these catheters lead to the development of the most common device-associated health care-associated infections (HAIs).[2–4] No national registry of HAIs exists, so the number of patients who suffer such complications is unknown. Analyses based on several data sets, however, including those from the Centers for Disease Control and Prevention (CDC) National Healthcare Safety Network (formerly the National Nosocomial Infections Surveillance system) and the American Hospital Association, all suggest that at least 500,000 health care–associated urinary tract infections (HA-UTIs) occur each year in US hospitals in the 5 million patients who have such catheters inserted.

Furthermore, these infections represent approximately one-third of all HAIs. Fortunately, the morbidity of HA-UTIs does not seem to create significant risk of death; these same data sources estimate that approximately 2.3% of these HAIs contribute to patient death, a rate lower than for any other type of HAI studied. The CDC reports that older age and increased severity of illness may contribute to the risk of death from HA-UTIs.[2–4] HA-UTIs are also recognized as one of the most frequent causes of bacteremia, second only to central venous catheters,[5] a conclusion disputed by some experts who found that HA-UTIs rarely contributed to bacteremia in their study

Infection Prevention & Control Department, NYU Langone Medical Center, New York, NY 10016, USA
E-mail address: steven.bock@nyumc.org

Perioperative Nursing Clinics 5 (2010) 449–456
doi:10.1016/j.cpen.2010.09.003
1556-7931/10/$ – see front matter © 2010 Elsevier Inc. All rights reserved.

of nearly 1500 hospitalized patients.[6] In the long-term care setting, HA-UTIs are the most common cause of bacteremia.[7]

The overwhelming consensus of expert opinion and many studies shows that the indwelling urinary catheter is the fundamental cause of urinary tract infections (UTIs).[2–4,8,9] Along with the presence of a catheter, many studies have shown that additional risk factors can lead to urinary catheter–associated UTIs (CAUTIs). These include duration of catheterization of at least 7 days; female gender, probably in large part due to the significantly shorter urethral length; insertion of the catheter outside of the operating room; having an infection at a different body site; chronic medical conditions, in particular those that may be immunosuppressive, such as diabetes mellitus and end-stage renal disease; malnutrition; use of the catheter simply for recording urinary output; failure to maintain a closed drainage system; and failure to keep the catheter collection bag below the level of the bladder (**Table 1**).[3,4,10] Severe neutropenia and frequent diarrhea may also be important CAUTI risk factors affecting a small subset of catheterized patients.

PATHOGENESIS OF CAUTI

The perineum is normally contaminated with large numbers of bacteria, often originating from the colon. As a result, the organisms that cause CAUTI are typically the same species found on these body surfaces. These include Enterobacteriaceae, such as *Escherichia, Klebsiella, Enterobacter*, and *Proteus* as well as *Pseudomonas*, along with streptococci, such as *Enterococcus*. *Candida* and *Staphylococci* are also recognized uropathogens (**Table 2**).[3–5,10] The gram-negative bacteria responsible for CAUTI account for up to approximately two-thirds of all such infections, with one species (*Escherichia*) accounting for at least one-third of all CAUTIs.

Contamination of the bladder can occur by both intraluminal and extraluminal passage of microbes and improper or inadequate care practices can allow either or both to occur.[3,4,8,9] Although a catheter can allow for the entry of bacteria and yeasts by both routes, the precise mechanism of bladder contamination is different. Intraluminal contamination typically occurs when the outward flow of urine from the bladder to the collection device or bag beyond the catheter is interrupted, blocked, or reversed. The drainage bag often serves as an important reservoir of bacteria or yeast due to the ability of bacteria to replicate rapidly in this environment. Microbial entry into the catheter system can occur by accidental contamination of the catheter's drainage port by bacteria in the environment or the catheter-tubing junction when the two are separated by accident or to collect a specimen.

The gram-negative coliform bacteria are often in a patient's periurethral environment and bedding and are the typical organisms that cause UTI via the intraluminal

Table 1 Risk factors for CAUTI	
Patient-Centered CAUTI Risk Factors	**Clinician-Centered CAUTI Risk Factors**
Female gender	Duration of catheterization ≥7 days
Infection at a different body site	Insertion of catheter outside the operating room
Diabetes mellitus	Failure to maintain a closed drainage system
End-stage renal disease	Catheterization only for urine output measurement
Malnutrition	Failure to keep collection bag below the bladder

Other possible contributing risk factors may include severe neutropenia and chronic diarrhea. *Data from* Refs.[4,10]

Table 2
Microorganisms responsible for causing CAUTI

Gram Negative Bacteria	Gram-Positive Bacteria	Yeasts
Escherichia	Enterococcus (fecalis/faecium)	Candida albicans
Klebsiella	Coagulase-negative staphylococci	Candida glabrata
Enterobacter	Staphylococcus aureus	Candida tropicalis
Proteus		
Pseudomonas		

Data from Refs.[4,5,10]

route.[4,6] The crystals of urine that may become deposited on the interior surface of a catheter can form a complex matrix that can then harbor bacteria that have been introduced to the system via the extraluminal route, making eradication difficult.[5] Fortunately, the intraluminal route of microbial entry may be easy to prevent with appropriate patient care practices although the fact that CAUTI is an ongoing problem may suggest poor patient care practices occur regularly. Changing the catheter and drainage tubing may offer some benefit for patients who have CAUTI but no evidence-based practices for such changes have been determined.[10]

In general, the extraluminal mechanism is considered the more likely route of bladder contamination.[4,6,8] Extraluminal movement of germs from outside the body to the bladder can initially occur when a catheter is inserted due to improper cleansing of the meatal area or contamination of the catheter during the insertion process.[5] For most patients, extraluminal microbial entry via a urinary catheter is a more gradual process that involves growth of the microbes along a catheter's external surface, often within the complex matrix of extrabacterial or fungal material, known as a biofilm. This biofilm often starts to develop shortly after a catheter is inserted, growing in a retrograde fashion, that is, from outside the body toward the bladder. The bacteria in a biofilm are often relatively immobilized by the proteins and other microscopic structures of the biofilm. They gradually become liberated from this layer, however, leading to free bacteria that can cause bladder infection. Increasing manipulation and movement of a catheter can cause release of bacteria from a biofilm into the bladder or into the urethral mucosa that may be irritated by the presence of the catheter.[5,11]

One consequence of extraluminal biofilm-related CAUTI is that women, who have anatomically shorter urethras, suffer more CAUTIs than men. Candida and gram-positive organisms, especially *Enterococci*, are the most common microbes associated with biofilm development; when such organisms are found to cause CAUTI, it can be presumed that the biofilm on the catheter's surface is the mechanism of microbial entry. Prevention of biofilm-related CAUTI may be more difficult to achieve and is the subject of much research.[4,9]

Biofilm formation prevention may be at least partially achieved by using catheters coated with antimicrobial chemicals, such as silver-based compounds; chlorhexidine, which is a commonly used antiseptic agent; or nitrofuranzone, an antibiotic compound. Many studies have sought to demonstrate benefit from using treated urinary catheters to reduce the risks of CAUTI but many have produced mixed results. This literature has failed to generate firm recommendations for the use of treated catheters.[3–6,10] Some experts instead suggest the consideration of catheter replacement in place of or before antibiotic therapy in patients with CAUTI in an effort to overcome biofilm-related CAUTI.[5] Again, the evidence for such a strategy is less than compelling.

CAUTI is preceded by bacteriuria or candiduria. Bacteriuria occurs when microbial colony counts in the bladder reach just 100 or 1000 microorganisms (colony-forming units) per milliliter, which can take just a day or two from the time of catheter insertion. Experts estimate that the risk of bacteriuria occurs at approximately 5% per day and that all patients who have catheters for 30 days have bacteriuria at the level of at least 100,000 colony-forming units (CFUs) per milliliter of urine. Most definitions of CAUTI include bacteria or yeast counts at greater than 10^5 CFU/mL, although most patients with this level of bladder contamination do not have symptoms and do not warrant treatment.

The administration of antimicrobial drugs may slow the initial development of bacteriuria, but it does not prevent the development of bacteriuria or CAUTI and instead usually serves to promote the growth of organisms that are drug resistant.[3–5,12] One expert suggests that despite these risks, prophylactic antibiotic administration with catheterization may benefit select patient populations, such as solid organ transplant or neutropenic patients.[7]

Although CAUTI can be symptomatic, most patients with CAUTI are symptom-free. It is believed that two main reasons lead to an absence of symptoms. Studies of non-catheterized patients with symptomatic UTI reveal that irritation of the urethra by the presence of bacteria and the distension of the bladder walls by contaminated urine are responsible for the dysuria, pyuria, and abdominal tenderness that are associated with such infections. In catheterized patients, the bladder is continuously drained and the catheter itself prevents contact between the bacteria and the urethral lining. The proteinaceous nature of the biofilm on a catheter's exterior serves as a shield to protect the bacteria within the biofilm from actual contact with the urethral epidermis. The relative value of various symptoms (eg, pyuria, fever, and suprapubic tenderness) in diagnosing CAUTI is the subject of much study and debate. Most experts agree, however, that a combination of symptoms and urine culture results is needed to define CAUTI[3,5,12–14] The strategies of treating CAUTI are beyond the scope of this article.

CATHETER USE IN THE SURGICAL PATIENT

The 2009 *Perioperative Standards and Recommended Practices* guidelines from the Association of periOperative Registered Nurses[11] contain no standards pertaining to when to use or remove urinary catheters. The urinary drainage needs of surgical patients receive scant attention in these guidelines, appearing merely in a list of physiologic parameters requiring pre-, peri-, or postoperative nursing assessment. There is discussion of neither the need for mechanical drainage of the bladder nor standards for the provision of such drainage. However, insertion and care of urinary catheters is a basic nursing skill covered in all major nursing texts.

Instead, the use of catheters seems to be subject merely to the traditional practice standards established at any given surgical center or hospital, apart from information and analyses gleaned from carefully controlled studies or even published expert opinion. Consequently, the use of an indwelling urinary catheter in patients undergoing surgery can vary substantially from hospital to hospital. More surprising, perioperative urinary catheter use may vary within an individual facility, depending on which surgeon is performing the procedure.[15]

Fortunately, there is some expert consensus that may help determine when patients should be catheterized for a surgical procedure. The CDC offers some indirect guidance for the use of urinary catheters to prevent surgery-related complications, stating,[3] "urinary retention in patients without catheters was specifically seen following urogenital surgeries." They concurrently offer the imprecise advice that "for operative patients, low-quality evidence suggested a benefit of avoiding urinary catheterization,"[3] contradicting the use of urinary drainage during surgery. These experts provide no insight into when such drainage may be beneficial or how to achieve such drainage while minimizing the infectious risks associated with catheter use.

Other authorities provide some guidance, suggesting that urinary catheters are indicated in some surgical settings.[7] Urinary drainage during surgery is known to help prevent certain complications from occurring during or in the first 24 to 48 hours after surgery. An undrained bladder can lead to increased physical and psychological stress for the patient. It can also lead to physiologic complications, including elevated blood pressure and heart rate. A distended bladder may create anatomic difficulties during some surgeries, causing pressure on other structures being manipulated during the procedure.[16] Patients undergoing prolonged (eg, at least 3–4 hours), cardiac, intracranial, or major abdominal surgery are often considered appropriate candidates for perioperative urinary catheterization. Patients who intraoperatively receive substantial fluid administration or diuretic therapy and those who are expected to experience large fluid shifts or have congestive heart failure also should have mechanical urinary drainage (**Table 3**).[3,4,17]

Several experts agree with the CDC recommendation that catheters generally be avoided in surgical patients or at least removed as soon as possible after the surgery.[3,4,10] Several small studies demonstrate that for surgeries where catheters are commonly used, equal patient outcomes with fewer UTIs or other urological complications occurred with earlier than normal catheter removal was practiced.

Italian researchers found that catheter removal immediately after hysterectomy when patients were still in the operating room yielded the fewest postoperative UTIs. Patients who had their catheters removed 6 hours after surgery had fewer UTIs than those who had their catheters removed 12 hours after surgery. The first cohort of patients also had the shortest hospital stays. Although this study was too small for statistical confirmation of the findings, the differences between each group were large.[18]

Another small study found no difference in the rates of postoperative urinary retention requiring reinsertion of an indwelling urinary catheter when the catheter was removed either 1, 3, or even 5 days after major pelvic surgery. The investigators conclude that early catheter removal does not predispose patients to needing recatheterization, which means early catheter removal may reduce catheter-associated complications, such as CAUTI.[19]

A larger study followed patients who underwent major thoracic and/or abdominal surgery and had thoracic spinal anesthesia, which is known to create significant risk for postoperative urinary retention. Patients were randomized either to have catheters removed the morning after surgery, while their epidural anesthesia was still being administered, or to have catheters removed only when the epidural was discontinued, usually 3 to 5 days after the surgery. Not surprisingly, the patients who had their catheters

Table 3 Surgical settings for appropriate perioperative urinary drainage	
Types of Surgery	**Procedure- or Patient-Related Circumstances**
Prolonged surgery (at least 3–4 hours)	Substantial intraoperative fluid administration
Cardiac surgery	Intraoperative diuretic therapy
Intracranial surgery	Anticipated large fluid shifts
Major abdominal surgery	Measuring urine output during surgery
Surgical repair of the genitourinary tract	Underlying congestive heart failure

Data from Refs.[3,4,17]

removed the morning after surgery had far fewer UTIs and significantly shorter hospital stays. Although they had a small increase in the need for intermittent catheterization to address postoperative urinary retention, this difference was not statistically significant from those patients who had catheters removed when the epidural was stopped.[15]

One institution identified an unusual complication from mechanical urinary drainage resulting in extreme pain and bladder spasm, termed Carignan syndrome. Prolonged surgery in men, where the catheter, drainage tubing, or collection bag was not adequately secured, led to increased catheter traction and resulted in migration of the inflated catheter balloon into the upper portion of the urethra. As patients were awakened from anesthesia, the excruciating symptoms were immediately reported. Although appropriate catheter securement corrected the problem, avoiding catheterization would have achieved the same result.[20]

The insertion and maintenance of indwelling catheters is also a practice subject to substantial variation. Depending on the staffing and work practice patterns of each surgical facility, catheters may be inserted by a physician, a physician's assistant, a certified surgical technician, a certified nurse anesthetist, or a registered nurse. How each type of health care worker inserts a urinary catheter depends on when and where the practitioner was trained. Complicating the variable of who inserts the catheter is which device is used and how it is inserted.

Most experts agree that a closed drainage system, where the catheter is preattached to a drainage tubing and collection bag is an imperative standard of care. Sterile technique for the insertion, using at least sterile gloves and sterile catheter/urethral lubricant and avoiding contaminating a catheter while performing the insertion, is also necessary to minimize the risk of CAUTI. Likewise, broad consensus exists to support keeping the drainage bag below the level of the bladder and avoid contamination of the collection bag drain spigot.[3,4,7–9,13]

Authorities disagree, however, on how to prepare the meatal site for catheter insertion; use of an antiseptic solution may not lead to reduced UTI risk compared with using simple soap and water cleansing. Whether or not to use an antiseptic-treated catheter, too, is subject to extensive debate in the literature, with little conclusive evidence supporting its use, especially in patients who are catheterized for up to 7 days. Further, catheter securement practices vary with no firm recommendation from the CDC.[3,4,7–9,13]

Perioperative staff may not routinely play a role in patient or urinary catheter management after surgery but knowledge of how patients are managed in order to minimize the risk of CAUTI is important. Patient education may be provided before the start of surgery to encourage postoperative care that minimizes the dependence on the urinary catheter. Staff in a postanesthesia care unit setting can play an role in assessing whether or not a catheter can be removed even before patients are discharged to the regular nursing unit. Surgical nursing leadership can play a vital role in establishing and maintaining practice standards that optimize the use of urinary catheters for those patients who truly need them.

SUMMARY

Currently there are no standards from any recognized perioperative authority as to which patients should receive perioperative mechanical urinary drainage or how long these catheters should remain in place after surgery. This absence of evidence-based practice is partly due to conflicting research findings on many aspects of urinary catheter care. Nonetheless, careful review of the existing guidelines from the CDC and other authorities may provide sufficient direction for surgical leaders to begin to form clear consensus statements regarding urinary perioperative care.

Future study into the development of catheters, drainage systems, and collection bags that resist the development of biofilms and the growth of microorganisms will undoubtedly help prevent CAUTIs. For perioperative team members, reducing the likelihood that a urinary catheter–associated infection develops depends on scrupulous attention to the aseptic and clean techniques for inserting and maintaining urinary catheters along with strict adherence to the timely removal of catheters. Most of all, developing and following guidelines to eliminate the need to use urinary catheters in most surgical patients will help prevent the greatest number of CAUTIs.

REFERENCES

1. Wikipedia. Foley Frederic. Available at: http://en.wikipedia.org/wiki/Frederic_Foley#Foley.27s_catheter. Accesssed January 3, 2010.
2. Klevens RM, Edwards JR, Richards CL Jr, et al. Estimating health care-associated infections and deaths in U.S. hospitals, 2002. Public Health Rep 2007;122(2):160–6.
3. CDC. Guideline for prevention of catheter-associated urinary tract infections 2009. healthcare infection control practices advisory committee (HICPAC). p. 34. Available at: http://www.cdc.gov/ncidod/dhqp/dpac_uti_pc.html. Accessed March 1, 2010.
4. Maki DG, Tambyah PA. Engineering out the risk for infection with urinary catheters. Emerg Infect Dis 2001;7(2):342–7.
5. Trautner BW, Darouiche RO. Catheter-associated infections: pathogenesis affects prevention. Arch Intern Med 2004;164:842–50.
6. Tambyah P, Halvorson K, Maki D. Prospective study of pathogenesis of catheter-associated urinary tract infections. Mayo Clin Proc 1999;74(2):131–6.
7. Warren JW. Catheter-associated urinary tract infections. Infect Dis Clin North Am 1997;11(3):609–22.
8. Diana Parker D, Callan L, Harwood J, et al. Nursing interventions to reduce the risk of catheter-associated urinary tract infection part 1: catheter selection. J Wound Ostomy Continence Nurs 2009;36(1):23–34.
9. Willson M, Wilde M, Webb ML, et al. Nursing interventions to reduce the risk of catheter-associated urinary tract infection part 2: staff education, monitoring, and care techniques. J Wound Ostomy Continence Nurs 2009;36(2):137–54.
10. Ksycki MF, Namias N. Nosocomial urinary tract infection. Surg Clin North Am 2009;89:475–81.
11. Perioperative standards and recommended practices. Denver (CO): Association of peri-Operative Registered Nurses; 2009.
12. Tambyah P, Maki D. Catheter-associated urinary tract infection is rarely symptomatic: a prospective study of 1497 catheterized patients. Arch Intern Med 2000; 160:678–82.
13. Newman DK. The indwelling urinary catheter: principles for best practice. J Wound Ostomy Continence Nurs 2007;34(6):655–61.
14. Tambyah P, Maki D. The relationship between pyuria and infection in patients with indwelling urinary catheters: a prospective study of 761 patients. Arch Intern Med 2000;160:673–7.
15. Zaouter C, Kaneva P, Carli F. Less urinary tract infection by earlier removal of bladder catheter in surgical patients receiving thoracic epidural analgesia. Reg Anesth Pain Med 2009;34(6):542–8.
16. Ramakrishnan K, Mold JW. Urinary catheters: a review. The internet. J Fam Pract 2005;3(2):2. Available at: http://www.ispub.com/journal/the_internet_journal_of_

family_practice/volume_3_number_2_16/article_printable/urinary_catheters_a_review.html. Accessed February 28, 2010.

17. Morgan GE Jr, Mikhail MS, Murray MJ. Urinary output (article 6). clinical anesthesiology, 4e. Available at: http://www.accessanesthesiology.com/content/886893. Accesssed January 3, 2010.

18. Alessandri F, Mistrangelo E, Lijol D, et al. A prospective, randomized trial comparing immediate versus delayed catheter removal following hysterectomy. Acta Obstet Gynecol 2006;85:716–29.

19. Zmora O, Madbouly K, Tulchinsky H, et al. Urinary bladder catheter drainage following pelvic surgery-is it necessary for that long? Dis Colon Rectum 2010; 53(3):321–6.

20. Nelson L, Carignan N. Catheter securement devices; a canadian case study. Surg Serv Manag 2000;6(8):9–10.

Surgical Skin Antisepsis

Robert Garcia, BS, MT (ASCP), CIC

KEYWORDS

- Surgical site infection • Skin antisepsis • Antiseptics
- Preoperative bathing • Preoperative showering
- Surgical scrub • Decolonization • Chlorhexidine gluconate

Skin antisepsis is a standard procedure performed thousands of times each day in countless health care facilities, particularly involving surgical patients. Three principle periods in which skin antisepsis is often performed on the surgical patient include a preoperative period whereby the patient typically applies the decolonizing agent after a bath or shower, during the surgical scrub of the skin done before incision, and as a decolonization measure as may occur when the patient is in a surgical intensive care unit (ICU).

Despite the acceptance and wide-spread use of topical antiseptics in various combinations and concentrations, basic questions such as which antiseptic is most effective in reducing surgical site infection risk appear to remain unanswered.

Most antiseptic solutions used for degerming skin in the United States contain one or a combination of three active ingredients: alcohol, chlorhexidine gluconate (CHG), or iodine.[1,2] Alcohol's principle antimicrobial activity is achieved by denaturing bacterial proteins. Concentrations of alcohol over 60% are most effective. Both gram-negative and gram-positive bacteria, including methicillin-resistant *Staphylococcus aureus* (MRSA) and vancomycin-resistant *Enterococcus* (VRE), are highly susceptible against alcohols. Alcohol's greatest advantage may be its ability to provide a quick germicidal kill. However, alcohol lacks any sustained activity (ie, it has little if any residual effect after drying).

CHG is characterized by good broad-spectrum activity against both gram-positive and gram-negative bacteria. One apparent benefit of using CHG is the ability to remain active even in the presence of organic material, including blood. This is particularly important when considering preoperative skin preparation. CHG also has substantial residual activity, a key advantage when a principle goal is to maximally reduce bacterial growth over extended periods of time, such as after surgery.[3,4]

The mechanism of germicidal activity of iodine-containing products is characterized by iodine's ability to bind with amino and unsaturated fatty acids, which leads to disruption of protein synthesis and cell membrane destruction. Most iodine-containing solutions currently manufactured are iodophors, which include a high molecular

No funding support to report.
Enhanced Epidemiology, PO Box 211, Valley Stream, NY 11580, USA
E-mail address: rgarciaicp@aol.com

Perioperative Nursing Clinics 5 (2010) 457–477
doi:10.1016/j.cpen.2010.07.004
1556-7931/10/$ – see front matter © 2010 Published by Elsevier Inc.

weight polymer carrier. The polymer allows for greater solubility and sustained release of iodine. Iodine compounds provide good activity against gram-negative and gram-positive bacteria; however, activity is substantially reduced in the presence of organic substances including blood. Antibacterial effectiveness after application is low, with most studies demonstrating persistent activity ranging from 30 to 60 minutes.

GUIDELINES ON ANTISEPTIC INTERVENTIONS

Preoperative skin decolonization and surgical skin preparation are preventive issues addressed in three major guidelines published by several expert organizations (**Table 1**). The most recent issue of the Centers for Disease Control and Prevention's (CDC) Hospital Infection Control Practices Advisory Committee's (HICPAC) Guideline on Preventing Surgical Site Infection was released in 1999.[5] When addressing the subject of preoperative showering, the consensus of the HICPAC authors was that health organizations should establish programs whereby decolonization is incorporated into their infection prevention efforts. The main scientific support for this recommendation was based on a study that involved treatment of over 700 patients with two preoperative CHG showers. Results indicated that bacterial colony counts on skin were reduced ninefold.[6] Several other studies were cited,[7,8] including one trial that indicated maximum antiseptic concentrations were achieved with repeated antiseptic bathing applications.[9] HICPAC at the time of publication conceded that published studies on antiseptic bathing did not definitively demonstrate a reduction in surgical site infection (SSI) rates. It should be noted that the guideline is more than a decade old.

As to the issue of patient skin preparation before surgery, HICPAC stated that "no studies have adequately assessed comparative effects of these preoperative skin antiseptics on SSI risk in well-controlled, operation-specific studies." However, antiseptics commonly used for this purpose have been well studied, with alcohol having the most rapid acting bacteriostatic effect and chlorhexidine gluconate exhibiting the longest kill time (residual effect) after application (**Table 2**).

The Society for Healthcare Epidemiology of America (SHEA) and the Infectious Diseases Society of America (IDSA) also have published SSI preventive guidelines, released in 2008.[10] In addressing the need for preoperative bathing or showering, the authors came to the conclusion that there was insufficient evidence that such practices prevent SSI, and therefore the issue in their interpretation remains an unresolved one. This conclusion is wholly based on a single publication from the Cochrane Collaborative[11] in which the literature was extensively reviewed and analyzed and which has now been widely referenced in other surgical research. The lone statement on preoperative skin preparation recommends the "…use [of] an appropriate antiseptic agent" and is referenced by the HICPAC guideline. No specific antiseptic agent was recommended.

The recommendations published by the Association of Operating Room Nurses (AORN) concerning preoperative showering and antiseptic skin prepping are extensive and thorough.[12] AORN cites scientific evidence that CHG is most effective in reducing bacterial burden during preoperative showering, and specifically states that two applications should be used before surgery for maximizing bacteriostatic result. They also acknowledge that studies have not shown that preoperative showers have demonstrated reductions in SSIs. AORN goes on to further state that CHG should be rinsed off the skin to avoid potential skin irritation. However, no evidence is provided that skin sensitivities or even allergic reactions occur on any significant level. Subjects in the study by Edmiston,[13] some of whom had multiple applications of CHG without rinsing, experienced no skin reactions at all. Of the more than 800 patients who had CHG applied on a daily basis (average 5.7 days per patient) in the study by Bleasdale,[14] none were observed to have an adverse skin reaction.

AORN makes an important point when it recommends that highly contaminated areas, whether they are the central focus of the surgery or adjacent to the surgical site, should be prepared separately (using eg, an applicator, which is then discarded). A second applicator should then be used to prepare the additional surgical site. The antiseptic manufacturer's instructions on application and drying times should be followed. The current US Food and Drug Administration (FDA)-approved alcohol–chlorhexidine skin antiseptic product designed for surgical skin preparation requires repeated back-and-forth strokes for 30 seconds (dry areas such as abdomen) or 2 minutes for moist areas (eg, inguinal folds). This methodology allows for the deep penetration of the active ingredients into the upper layers of the skin.

Both the CDC and AORN make note of applying an antiseptic to the skin surface in concentric circles. Neither of the guidelines provides any supportive references for this statement. No studies have been published that compare methods of antiseptic application. However, when the basic structure of the skin is understood, it becomes apparent that scrubbing vigorously back and forth is necessary to achieve maximum contact between the active ingredient in the antiseptic solution and potential pathogenic bacteria.

Transient bacteria (ie, organisms that are most often acquired by health care workers during direct patient contact or during contact with a contaminated environment) reside on the topmost layer of skin, the superficial layer (10 to 20 μm thick). Resident flora, such as coagulase-negative staphylococci, are found in the next layer of skin, the epidermis (50 to 100 μm thick). Normal human skin contains billions of bacteria. The abdomen alone, a common surgical site, has bacterial counts that average 4×10^4 CFUs/cm²[2] Countless crevices, openings for the transfer of nutrients and waste, hair follicles, and other complex structures provide haven for bacteria. The combination of the sheer numbers of organisms and the complexity of skin structure make microorganisms, including resistant bacteria, difficult to remove. The application of an antiseptic from the inner to outer perimeter of the prepared area (ie, in concentric circles) in theory does not allow for maximum penetration into the upper skin layers, and therefore limits contact to very superficial bacteria. A study that reported poor penetration of chlorhexidine in layers of human skin samples required the investigator to place the antiseptic on the skin surface rather than scrub the solution into the skin before measurement.[15]

PREOPERATIVE SHOWERING

For over 30 years, health care facilities have established decolonizing programs as part of their presurgical regimens in the belief that such actions would decrease the risk of either resident or transient bacteria becoming pathogenic and causing postsurgical infection as may occur when skin in incised and manipulated. The value of implementing preventive initiatives such as preoperative bathing or showering with skin antiseptics, particularly CHG, has come into question since the publication of a Cochrane Collaboration review on the subject.[11] The authors of the review conducted a broad search of the scientific literature, which originally identified 43 articles for potential inclusion. Studies were included in the final review if they were randomized, controlled trials, if they specifically examined the effectiveness of an antiseptic solution(s) used for preoperative bathing or showering, and if they reported the primary

Table 1
Key organization recommendations on preoperative decolonization and preoperative skin preparation

Organization, Guideline, Publication Year of Most Recent Guideline	Recommendation on Preoperative Showering	Guideline Category	Recommendation on Preoperative Skin Preparation	Guideline Category
HICPAC, Guideline for Prevention of Surgical Site Infection, 1999	Require patients to shower or bathe with an antiseptic agent on a least the night before the operative day	IB	Use an appropriate antiseptic agent for skin preparation. Apply preoperative antiseptic skin preparation in concentric circles moving toward the periphery. The prepared area must be large enough to extend the incision or create new incisions or drain sites, if necessary.	IB II
SHEA/IDSA, Strategies to Prevent Surgical Site Infections in Acute Care Hospitals, 2008	Several studies have examined the utility of preoperative showers, but none have definitively proven that they decrease SSI risk. A recent Cochrane review evaluated the evidence for preoperative bathing or showering with antiseptics for SSI prevention. Six randomized controlled trials evaluating the use of 4% chlorhexidine gluconate were included in the analysis, with no clear evidence of benefit noted.	Unresolved issue	Wash and clean skin around incision site; use an appropriate agent	A-II
AORN, 2010	Patients undergoing open Class I surgical procedures below the chin should have two preoperative showers with CHG before surgery, when appropriate. 4% CHG is more effective than povidone–iodine or soap, and more than one shower is necessary to achieve maximum antiseptic effectiveness. Although there is sufficient evidence of the effectiveness of two CHG showers to reduce microbial counts, there is insufficient research to definitively link this decrease in microbial count to a reduction I SSI rate.	NA	The skin around the surgical site should be free of soil, debris, exudates, and transient microorganisms to minimize contamination of the surgical wound before application of the antiseptic skin preparation. The antiseptic agent should be applied to the skin over the surgical site and surrounding area in a manner to minimize contamination, preserve skin integrity, and prevent tissue damage. When not part of the surgical procedure, a highly contaminated site (eg, anus, colostomy) should be isolated from the area to be prepared. (isolating the contaminated area confines and contains microorganisms away from the surgical site).	NA

Following each preoperative shower, the skin should be thoroughly rinsed, dried with a fresh, clean, dry towel, and the patient should don clean clothing. Rinsing the skin removes residual CHG that may cause skin irritation. Patients undergoing surgery on the head should be instructed or assisted to perform two preoperative shampoos with 4% CHG before surgery to reduce the number of microorganisms and subsequent contamination of the surgical site.	Application of the skin antiseptic should progress from the incision site to the periphery of the surgical site. In most surgical procedures, the incision site is in close proximity to anatomic areas with high microbial counts (eg, laparotomy incision/umbilicus/groin; neck/mouth/nares; ankle/toes; shoulder/axilla; hand/fingernails). Progressing from the incision site to the periphery prevents reintroducing microorganisms from these areas into the incision site. When using a commercially available applicator, refer to the manufacturer's instructions to ensure uniform distribution of the antiseptic. If a highly contaminated area is part of the procedure, the area with a lower bacterial count is prepared first, followed by the area of higher contamination, as opposed to working from the incision site toward the periphery. When prepping the anus or vagina or stoma, sinus, ulcer, or open wound, the sponge should be applied once to that area and then discarded. The antiseptic agent should remain in place for the full time suggested by the manufacturer's written recommendations.

HICPAC Category IB = strongly recommended for implementation and supported by some experimental, clinical, or epidemiologic studies and strong theoretical rationale.

HICPAC Category II = suggested for implementation and supported by suggestive clinical or epidemiologic studies or theoretical rationale.

SHEA/IDSA Category A-II = good evidence to support a recommendation for use/evidence from ≥1 well-designed clinical trial, without randomization; from cohort or case-control analytic studies (preferably from > 1 center); from multiple time series; or from dramatic results from uncontrolled experiments.

Abbreviations: AORN, Association of Operating Room Nurses; CHG, chlorhexidine gluconate; HICPAC, Hospital Infection Control Practices Advisory Committee; IDSA, Infectious Disease Society of North America; NA, not applicable (AORN does not categorize recommendations in the Perioperative Standards and Recommended Practices publication); SHEA, Society for Healthcare Epidemiology of America; SSI, surgical site infection.

Table 2
Mechanism and spectrum of activity of antiseptic agents commonly used for preoperative skin preparation

Agent	Mechanism of Action	Gram-positive Bacteria	Gram-negative Bacteria	Mtb	Fungi	Virus	Rapidity of Action	Residual Activity	Toxicity	Uses
Alcohol	Denature proteins	E	E	G	G	G	Most rapid	None	Drying, volatile	SP, SS
Chlorhexidine	Disrupt cell membrane	E	G	P	F	G	Intermediate	E	Ototoxicity, keratitis	SP, SS
Iodine/Iodophors	Oxidation/substitution by free iodine	E	G	G	G	G	Intermediate	Minimal	Absorption from skin with possible toxicity, skin irritation	SP, SS

Abbreviations: E, excellent; F, fair; G, good; Mtb, *Mycobacterium tuberculosis*; P, poor; SP, skin preparation; SS, surgical scrubs.

Modified from Centers for Disease Control and Prevention. Hospital Infection Control Practices Advisory Committee. Guideline for prevention of surgical site infections. Atlanta (Georgia): Centers for Disease Control and Prevention; 1999.

outcome of surgical site infection. Seven trials[8,16-21] met the inclusion criteria; a summary of study findings is found in **Table 3**.

The conclusions reached by the Cochrane review on published studies addressing the effectiveness of CHG as a preoperative showering antiseptic in preventing SSIs appear on the surface to be accurate (ie, the authors conclude [mainly based on their analysis that two of the reviewed studies were of high quality] that there is no statistically significant reduction in surgical site infections when using chlorhexidine-based solutions during preoperative bathing).

The question arises as to why CHG would have been mostly ineffective in the these studies since CHG has been shown in many randomized, controlled studies to be effective in reducing bacterial infection in a various clinical applications and configurations, including surgical hand scrubs, skin preparation for intravascular insertions, oropharyngeal hygiene, and as a topical skin application for reducing infections, particularly in ICUs.[4,22-26] The principle reason that most of the reviewed studies failed to show any significant reductions in surgical site infection was clarified and described in a well-designed and innovative study published in 2008. Edmiston and colleagues[13] speculated that levels of CHG sufficient to reach minimal inhibitory concentrations (MICs) of the most common SSI pathogens could not be achieved in the cited studies, because CHG was rinsed off the skin during the bathing/showering process before the surgical operations. A modified method of application and use of a timed schedule followed by CHG concentration measurements were incorporated into the new study methodology. Bacterial cultures were taken from each study subject and determinations made for the CHG MIC for each staphylococcal isolate identified.

The main study was conducted in two parts. Ten subjects in a preliminary study were given a 4 oz bottle of antiseptic solution containing 4% CHG with no specific instructions for application technique or duration of exposure. This scenario reflected many of the studies in the Cochrane review. Subjects returned within a set time period (2–3 hours after showering) to determine CHG concentrations on the skin.

The randomized study consisted of three groups, each group consisting of 20 subjects. The study initially had subjects in three groups apply an antiseptic either in the evening, morning, or evening and morning. Subgroup A subjects used a 4% CHG-containing soap. Subjects were instructed to apply the solution with a clean washcloth, covering all body parts except the face and scalp. Subjects were instructed not to rinse the solution off; a second application was to be performed making sure that arms and legs (including the antecubital and popliteal fossas) and abdomen (including the umbilicus) once again were covered. After the second application, the solution was to remain on the skin for 2 minutes, rinsed off and the skin towel dried.

A 7-day washout period was initiated between the two subgroup interventions. In subgroup B, the 60 volunteers were required to shower using nonmedicated soap or body wash. After towel drying, the subjects scrubbed arms, legs, and the entire abdominal surface with three 2% CHG-impregnated cloths, one for each area. Skin was allowed to dry for a few minutes before dressing. Rinsing off of the solution was not to be done. Time of application was recorded, and subjects reported to a laboratory on a set time basis for sampling to determine CHG concentrations.

Sixty-one staphylococcal strains were isolated from the site cultures on the 10 volunteers in the pilot study. The MIC of CHG, which would inhibit the growth of 90% of the staphylococcal skin isolates (ie, MIC_{90}), was determined to be 4.8 ppm.

Table 3
Summary of studies examining the use of skin antiseptics during preoperative bathing or showering on surgical site infections

Author/ Year	Number of Subjects	Types of Surgery	Comparative Agents	Regimen	Patient Instructions	Definition of Infection	Time Frame for Determining SSI	Rate of SSI
Byrne 1992	3733	General (includes clean and potentially infected surgeries)	4% CHG (Hibiclens/ Riohex) detergent solution vs placebo (same detergent without CHG)	Showered on admission, the night before surgery and the morning of surgery	Groups: (1) 4% CHG: written instructions (2) Placebo: written instructions	Presence of pus	During hospitalization and for 6 weeks after discharge	(1) CHG group: 256/1754 (14.6%) (2) Placebo group: 272/1735 (15.7%)
Hayek 1987	2015	General	4% CHG (Hibiscus/ Riohex) detergent solution vs placebo (same detergent without CHG) 4% CHG (Hibiscus) vs bar soap	Shower or bath on day before and morning of operation	Groups: (1) 4% CHG: instruction card provided (2) Placebo: instruction card provided[a] (3) Bar soap: no instructions provided	Presence of pus from wound or erythema or swelling considered greater than expected	During hospitalization and for 6 weeks after discharge	(1) CHG group: 62/689 (9.0%) (2) Placebo group: 83/700 (11.7%) (3) Bar soap group: 80/626 (12.8%)
Earnshaw, 1989	66	Vascular reconstruction	4% CHG (Hibiscrub) vs bar soap	All patients had 2 baths	Groups: (1) 4% CHG: paint entire body with undiluted 4% CHG followed by rinsing (2) Soap: no specific instructions provided	Presence of pus	Reviewed patients twice weekly until discharge	(1) CHG group: 8/31 (26%) (2) Nonmedicated soap: 4/35 (11.4%)
Randell, 1983	93	Vasectomy	4% CHG (Hibiscrub) vs bar soap Chlorhexidine with no shower or bath	(1) q preoperative shower with 4% CHG (2) 1 shower with normal soap (3) No shower		Presence of pus or discharge of serous fluid	7 days	(1) CHG group: 12/32 (37.5%) (2) Soap: 10/30 (33.3%) (3) No shower: 9/32 (28.1%)

Surgical Skin Antisepsis   465

Study	N	Surgery type	Intervention	Special application instructions	Outcome definition	Follow-up	Results
Rotter, 1988	2813	General, orthopedic, vascular	4% CHG (Hibiclens/Riohex) detergent solution vs placebo (same detergent without CHG)	All patients had 2 showers, 1 on day before and 1 on the day of surgery (1) 50 mL of 4% CHG for each shower (2) Placebo	Inflammation of the surgical wound with discharge of pus	3 weeks	(1) CHG group: 37/1413 (2.6%) (2) Placebo group: 33/1400 (2.4%)
Wihlborg, 1987	1530	Biliary tract, inguinal hernia, or breast surgery	Chlorhexidine full body bathing vs localized washing (ie, restricted to the part of the body to be subjected to surgery [CHG used in both arms of study]) Chlorhexidine with no shower or bath	(1) Patients washed entire body with CHG on day before surgery using 2 consecutive applications followed by rinsing under the shower (2) Washed only part of body targeted for surgery with CHG soap (3) No CHG wash	Presence of pus	During hospitalization and among those returning for an outpatient visit	(1) CHG on entire body group: 9/541 (1.7%) (2) CHG on portion of body group: 23/552 (4.2%) (3) No CHG group: 20/437 (4.6%)
Veiga, 2009	150	Plastic	4% CHG (Hibiclens/Riohex) detergent solution vs placebo (same detergent without CHG) Chlorhexidine with no shower or bath	(1) Shower with liquid-based detergent containing 4% chlorhexidine (2) Shower with the same liquid based detergent, without CHG (3) No preoperative showering instructions were given	Patients in groups 1 and 2 were asked to rinse thoroughly, lather with the antiseptic, rinse, lather and rinse again	CDC definitions	30 days	(1) CHG group: 1/50 (2) Detergent group: 1/50 (3) No shower group: 0/50

Abbreviations: CDC, Centers for Disease Control and Prevention; CHG, chlorhexidine gluconate; SSI, surgical site infection.
[a] 5 months into study, the placebo was found to have antibacterial properties and was changed.

Data on group characteristics and CHG skin concentrations measured in each group are included in **Table 4**.

The results indicated that for subjects in subgroup A, the concentration of 4% CHG soap on the skin after initial application (no rinse), reapplication (allowing to remain on skin for a 2-minute interval), then rinsing and drying, rose steadily from group 1 through group 3. For subjects in subgroup B (2% CHG cloth), the concentration of CHG rose among the same groups. However, the CHG concentrations were significantly higher in the subgroup B volunteers (ie, those who applied the CHG using an impregnated cloth).

The study provides several key insights, all with potentially significant impact on the occurrence of SSI[1]:

CHG even when applied in a nonoptimal method followed by rinsing achieves concentrations that at a minimum are approximately five times sufficient to achieve 90% kill of the most common bacteria causing SSI[2]

CHG achieves highest concentrations when two applications are used (ie, a cumulative effect is observed as occurs when applied during the evening and in the morning)[3]

Gaps in skin concentration levels of CHG occurred when applied as a liquid poured onto a wash cloth (subgroup A)

Far greater levels of CHG were achieved when using the 2% CHG-impregnated cloth, leading one to speculate that deep scrubbing of the CHG into the skin allows for increased penetration of the antiseptic into crevices of the skin, areas where large numbers of bacteria exist.[3]

The requirement to not rinse the CHG off the skin ensures that extremely high concentrations of CHG will remain at the time of surgery. An evening and morning application of 2% CHG with the impregnated cloth without rinsing achieved levels greater than 363 times the MIC_{90}.

Edmiston and colleagues cite several design flaws in the studies contained in the Cochrane review that thus appear to contribute directly to faulty conclusions:

No routine standard of practice was applied to the implementation of the preoperative shower

Protocols did not exist as to the timed duration of the antiseptic showers

The surgical patients were highly heterogeneous, composed of various patients undergoing clean, clean-contaminated, and contaminated surgery

Compliance of the subjects to the study protocols was not reported in the studies.

PREOPERATIVE SKIN PREPPING

The Cochrane Collaborative also has reviewed the issue of whether the use of preoperative skin antiseptics prevents SSI.[27] The criteria limited selection to randomized controlled trials that evaluated preoperative skin antiseptics applied immediately before incision in clean surgical operations. After the initial searches, seven trials were judged to have met the inclusion criteria. It should be noted that the authors included studies in the final tally that tested the effectiveness of using iodine-impregnated incise drapes. Of the seven studies, only two compared antiseptic solutions that were painted or scrubbed onto the skin without use of antiseptic drapes in any of the comparative groups.[28,29]

In the study by Berry and colleagues,[28] 866 patients were randomized to receive skin prepping with povidone–iodine in 10% alcohol or chlorhexidine 0.5% in spirit

Table 4

Group treatment criteria and chlorhexidine gluconate concentrations, Edmiston study on 4% chlorhexidine gluconate soap versus 2% chlorhexidine gluconate cloth

Groups	Application Timeframe	Subgroup A Treatment	CHG Concentrations (ppm) for Subgroup A	Subgroup A Mean CHG Skin Concentrations over the MIC$_{90}$ of 4.8	Subgroup B Treatment	CHG Concentrations (ppm) for Subgroup B	Subgroup B Mean CHG Skin Concentrations over the MIC$_{90}$ of 4.8
1	Evening	4% CHG soap	17.2 to 31.6	5.1 times	2% CHG-impregnated cloth	361.5–443.8	90.2 times
2	Morning	4% CHG soap	51.6 to 119.6	17.8 times	2% CHG-impregnated cloth	907.0–1049.6	203.8 times
3	Evening and morning	4% CHG soap	101.4 to 149.6	>26.6 times	2% CHG-impregnated cloth	1484.6–2031.3	363.7 times

Abbreviations: CHG, chlorhexidine gluconate; MIC, minimum inhibitory concentration.

(Hibitane). Patients in each group received two applications of the corresponding antiseptic. Only data on 371 patients undergoing clean surgery were extracted. Significantly fewer patients developed an SSI when prepared with chlorhexidine (8 of 195 patients, 4.1%) than when skin was cleansed with povidone–iodine in 10% alcohol (28 of 176 patients, 15.9%).

In the second randomized trial, authored by Ellenhorn and colleagues,[29] patients undergoing abdominal surgery were divided into two groups, one to have a 5-minute skin preparation before surgery with 0.75% povidone–iodine scrub and 1% povidone–iodine paint compared with a second group that received 1% povidone–iodine paint. Follow-up was performed for only 30 days post-op. Infection rates for clean surgery were reported. Twice as many patients (8 of 34) developed SSI in the paint-only group as in the scrub and paint group (4 of 36).

The Cochrane review, first published in 2004 with edits in 2009, suggests that despite the publication of several randomized controlled studies, the question remains as to which antiseptic agent or combination of agents used for preparing skin surfaces before surgical incision may be superior in preventing SSIs. Until recently, no randomized controlled study had been published that attempted to determine the effect of using a specific preoperative skin antiseptic on reducing the occurrence of SSIs. In order to study this problem, Darouiche and colleagues[30] designed a 4-year trial in which patients scheduled to undergo clean-contaminated surgery at six university-affiliated hospitals in the United States would randomly undergo preoperative skin preparation by scrubbing with an applicator that contained a 70% alcohol with 2% CHG combination solution or by preoperatively scrubbing and painting the site with an aqueous solution of 10% povidone–iodine. The types of clean–contaminated surgeries performed were varied: colorectal, small intestinal, gastroesophageal, biliary, thoracic, gynecologic, or urologic operations. Operations that encountered substantial spillage or unusual contamination were not included in the study groups. Patients also were excluded from the trial if

They verbalized or demonstrated allergic reaction to chlorhexidine, alcohol, or iodophors

Any infection at or adjacent to the operative site was observed

Following the patient's outcomes for 30 days after the initial surgery date was not possible.

The main outcome measurement for this study was the occurrence of any surgical site infection within 30 days after surgery. In order to eliminate further bias, surgeons were not allowed to decide which skin antiseptic was to be used for their patient (ie, surgeons only became aware of which option was chosen at the postpreparation time after the patient was transported into the operating room. CDC criteria[1] were used to determine SSI. After the identification of an infection, the type of SSI was categorized as follows:

Superficial incisional infection (includes skin and subcutaneous tissue but not stitch-related abscesses)

Deep incisional infection (involves the fascia and muscle)

Organ–space infection (which involved any organ or space other than the incised layer of body wall that was opened or manipulated during the operation).

A long-standing concern in conducting accurate SSI surveillance and subsequent data analysis has been the gathering of information regarding signs and symptoms that may indicate a potential infection occurring after the discharge of the patient from the hospital.[31] The authors of this study attempted to enhance the surveillance mechanism for determining SSIs by initiating weekly phone contacts with the patients during the 30-day postsurgery period. Patients suspected of developing SSI were promptly scheduled for clinical evaluation to directly examine the operative site.

The results of the study were published in the New England Journal of Medicine in 2010. The number of patients enrolled in both arms of the study was sufficient to achieve 90% power to detect any significant difference between the groups (two-tailed significance level of 0.05 or less). After exclusion of some subjects because of pre-set criteria such as undergoing clean rather than clean–contaminated surgery, 391 patients who received chlorhexidine–alcohol skin preparation and 422 who were prepared using povidone–iodine were included in the final trial analysis. Comparison of the two study groups did not identify any significant differences in such factors as demographic characteristics, coexisting illnesses, use of systemic antibiotics, types of surgery, or the use of antibacterial preoperative showers.

The results of this well designed study give strong support that a combination product of 2% chlorhexidine with 70% alcohol is very effective in reducing the occurrence of SSI across a wide array of different types of surgeries. The overall rate of SSI was found to be significantly lower in the chlorhexidine–alcohol group (9.5%) as compared with patients in the group treated with povidone–iodine (16.1%) (**Table 5**). The relative risk of infection for all types of surgery in patients prepared with chlorhexidine–alcohol (39 SSIs) versus povidone–iodine (71 SSIs) was 0.59 (95% confidence interval [CI], 0.41–0.85). Use of a chlorhexidine–alcohol solution to prepare the skin at surgical sites was found to reduce SSI by 41% as compared with using aqueous povidone–iodine. When analysis was conducted to determine differences in infection rates between types of infections, it was shown that chlorhexidine–alcohol was associated with significant decrease in superficial incisional infections (relative risk [RR] 0.48, 95% CI, 0.41–0.85) and in deep incisional infections

Table 5
Proportion of patients with surgical site infection, according to type of infection (intention-to-treat population)

Type of Infection	Chlorhexidine-Alcohol (N = 409) Number (%)	Povidone–Iodine (N = 440) Number (%)	Relative Risk (95% CI)[a]	P Value[b]
Any surgical site infection	39 (9.5)	71 (16.1)	0.59 (0.41–0.85)	0.004
Superficial incisional infection	17 (4.2)	38 (8.6)	0.48 (0.28–0.84)	0.008
Deep incisional infection	4 (1.0)	13 (3.0)	0.33 (0.11–1.01)	0.05
Organ space infection	18 (4.4)	20 (4.5)	0.97 (0.52–1.80)	>0.99
Sepsis from surgical-site infection	11 (2.7)	19 (4.3)	0.62 (0.30–1.29)	0.26

[a] Relative risks are for chlorhexidine–alcohol as compared with povidone–iodine. The 95% confidence intervals were calculated with the use of asymptotic standard-error estimates.
[b] P values are based on Fisher's exact test.
From Darouiche RO, Wall MJ Jr, Itani KMF, et al. Chlorhexidine–alcohol versus povidone–iodine for surgical-site antisepsis. N Engl J Med 2010;362:23; with permission.

(RR 0.33, 95% CI, 0.11–1.01). However, no differences were detected between the groups in organ space infections (RR 0.62, 95% CI, 0.52–1.80) or in sepsis from SSI (RR 0.62, 95% CI, 0.30 –1.29).

Further analysis indicated two additional key findings. First, the risk for acquiring an SSI after surgery was found to be significantly longer when patients were treated with CHG than among those prepared with povidone–iodine. In all seven types of operations performed, rates of infection were shown to be lower in the CHG–alcohol group than in the povidone–iodine group in both the intention-to-treat analysis and the per-protocol analysis. Second, the study also reported significantly lower rates of infection in patients undergoing small intestinal surgery or abdominal surgery or who did not shower preoperatively and whose operative skin sites were prepared using chlorhexidine–alcohol. Multivariate logistic regression analysis identified use of povidone–iodine as a risk factor for developing SSI.

A commentary in the *New England Journal of Medicine* by Dr R. Wenzel places the results of this study in a new perspective:

"…The Darouiche study supports the value of a relatively inexpensive horizontal program, which was remarkably effective: the number of patients who would need to be treated to prevent one surgical site infection was found to be 17……In summary, the weight of evidence suggests that chlorhexidine–alcohol should replace povidone–iodine as the standard for preoperative surgical scrubs."[32]

DECOLONIZING PRACTICES

Patients awaiting surgery or immediately after surgery are often admitted to critical care units. Surgical critical care patients are at increased risk of becoming colonized with bacteria acquired after admission to the hospital, a significant portion of which may be multidrug resistant organisms (MROs). Such organisms are increasingly implicated as causing not only SSIs, but many other hospital-acquired infections also. Efforts to decolonize the skin of patients in health care settings has gained momentum in the United States and is being incorporated in many hospitals as part of their standard of care.

The evidence that daily application of antiseptics to the skin is effective in reducing bacterial colonization and subsequent infection is growing. Many hospitals that have established such programs have done so because of the limited success of infection control prevention strategies including hand washing. In one study conducted in a 21-bed ICU in a large Chicago hospital, the authors decided to test efforts directed at source control (ie, attempt to decolonize the skin of patients).[33] CHG was chosen as the decolonizing agent because of its known antibacterial spectrum and residual effect. Outcomes to be measured were acquisition of vancomycin-resistant *Enterococcus* (VRE) among patients and health care workers, as well as environmental contamination. Methods of bathing patients were altered during three consecutive study periods: soap and water basin baths (4 months), single-use disposable cloths impregnated with 2% CHG (5 months), and single-use cloths without CHG (5 months). Cultures for VRE were obtained from patients anticipated to be in the medical ICU for 3 or more days, with follow-up cultures taken every 1 to 2 days for those patients testing VRE-negative. More extensive culturing was taken on those whose cultures were positive. Environmental cultures were obtained from bed rails, pull sheets, and overbed tables each time cultures were taken from a VRE-positive patient. Hand cultures of health care workers were obtained randomly when exiting rooms of VRE-positive patients and before hand hygiene was performed.

Statistical analysis indicated that the risk for all parameters, including VRE acquisition by patients and health care workers, as well as environmental contamination, was not different when using either soap and water baths or baths using nonmedicated cloths but were significantly lower when chlorhexidine-impregnated cloths were used for bathing of patients (**Fig. 1**).

A second important study on the issue of decolonization and infection was conducted at the same Chicago hospital as the previously reviewed study by Vernon. However, the focus of this study was to ascertain the effect of using chlorhexidine-impregnated cloths on the incidence of primary bloodstream infection.[14] The study was designed as a 52-week, two-arm, crossover trial with intention-to-treat analysis. Two 11-bed ICUs were used as the study units. During an initial 28-week period, one hospital unit had all patients bathed daily with a 2% CHG-impregnated cloth while the second unit used daily bathing with soap and water. After a 2-week washout period, the interventions were reversed in the two units, again for another 28 weeks.

The results were dramatic. Patients undergoing CHG baths were significantly (61%) less likely to develop a primary bloodstream infection. There was no significant effect on other types of hospital-acquired infections (**Table 6**). Rates of central line-associated bacteremia were lower when CHG was used (6.4 bloodstream infections [BSIs] per 1000 catheter days) than when patients were bathed with plain soap and water (16.8 BSIs per 1000 catheter days). The study adds further support that reducing microbial burden with topical antiseptics such as CHG significantly lowers acquired infections, in this study both primary and catheter-associated infections.

A study comprising the effects of a CHG decolonizing program on patients for both MRO acquisition and bloodstream infection was published in 2009.[34] The trial by Climo and colleagues advances the notion that a CHG decolonization regimen reduces skin colonization and development of infection, particularly since the study took place in six ICUs at four academic medical centers. The ICUs were a mixture of medical, surgical, coronary, and cardiac care units. In an initial 6-month baseline period, all patients admitted to the ICUs were bathed daily using soap and water. During the second 6-month period, patients were cleansed with a prepared antiseptic

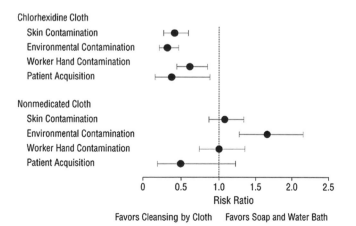

Fig. 1. Risk ratios for skin contamination and environmental or health care worker contamination or by patient acquisition of vancomycin-resistant enterococci (VRE). (*From* Vernon MO, Hayden MK, Trick WE, et al. Chlorhexidine gluconate to cleanse patients in a medical intensive care unit. Arch Intern Med 2006;166:309; with permission.)

Table 6
Comparison of incidence of infection by method of bathing patients and infection category

Infection Category	Bathing Method				Difference (95% CI)	P Value
	Soap and Water		2% CHG			
	Events	Rate[a]	Events	Rate[a]		
Primary BSI	22	10.4	9	4.1	6.3 (1.2 to 11)	.01
Contaminant	9	4.3	4	1.8	2.4 (−0.9 to 5.7)	.16
Clinical sepsis	9	4.2	16	7.2	−3.0 (−7.5 to 1.5)	.20
Urinary tract infection	17	8.0	13	5.9	2.1 (−2.8 to 7.1)	.41
Ventilator-associated pneumonia	15	6.8	18	7.8	−1.1 (−6.3 to 4.1)	.69
Secondary BSI	5	2.4	5	2.3	0 (−2.8 to 3.0)	.95
Clostridium difficile diarrhea	20	9.4	21	9.5	0 (−5.9 to 5.7)	.98

Abbreviations: BSI, bloodstream infection; CHG, chlorhexidine gluconate; CI, confidence interval.
[a] Rates are expressed per 1000 patient–days. There were 2119 patient–days in the soap and water arm and 2210 patient-days in the CHG arm.
Data From Bleadsdale SC, Trick WE, Gonzalez IM, et al. Effectiveness of chlorhexidine bathing to reduce catheter-associated bloodstream infections in medical intensive care unit patients. Arch Intern Med 2007;167:2073–79.

solution (4-oz bottle of 4% CHG mixed with warm water in a 6-qt basin). No other interventions aimed at MRO control or BSI elimination took place during the study periods.

The use of daily bathing patients with CHG resulted in a 25% decrease in the acquisition of MRSA. Bacteremias caused by MRSA were not affected, since few cases were seen in either of the groups. The effect on both VRE acquisition and bacteremia was more dramatic (**Table 7**). The VRE acquisition rate among patients treated with CHG declined by 45%, while rates of VRE bacteremia were observed to decrease significantly (78%) (**Fig. 2**). The authors note that a prompt reduction in the incidence of VRE followed the introduction of CHG bathing, observed as an immediate decrease of 1.44 cases per 1000 patient days.

Additional studies seem to support the elimination of soap and water bathing and substitution with CHG bathing to control bacterial colonization and subsequent infection.[35–37]

BEST PRACTICES FOR USE OF SURGICAL ANTISEPTICS

With the understanding of the necessary interaction between an antiseptic and the normal skin surface and the scientific information culled from many recently published studies, protocols written for the application of a surgical antiseptic should consider the following[12,38,39]:

The antiseptic manufacturer should clearly state on the label of the product a minimum of five criteria: active ingredient and concentration, area of skin coverage of a single applicator, method and duration of application, drying time, and precautionary statements (eg, potential flammability). If the manufacturer does not outline these requirements, consideration must be made to seek another antiseptic.

Table 7
Time series analysis of the results of introduction of daily chlorhexidine bathing on the incidence of MRSA and VRE colonization and bacteremia

Outcome Measure	Incidence Rate as Modeled at End of Intervention in the Absence of Chlorhexidine Bathing[a]	Observed Incidence Rate at End of Intervention[b]	Change in Incidence Rate Attributable to Introduction of Chlorhexidine Bathing (% Change)[c]
MRSA incidence	2.59	1.93	−0.66 (25%)
MRSA bacteremia	<0.1	<0.1	0 (0)
VRE incidence	3.34	1.83	−1.51 (45%)
VRE bacteremia	3.38	0.74	−2.64 (78%)

Abbreviation: MRSA, methicillin-resistant Staphylococcus aureus; VRE, vancomycin-resistant Enterococcus.

[a] Incidence rate (cases per 1000 patient–days) as modeled in time series analysis at the end of the intervention period based on level and secular trends observed during the baseline period in the absence of chlorhexidine bathing. This represents the expected value that would be observed had chlorhexidine bathing not been introduced.

[b] Modeled incidence rate (cases per 1000 patient–days) observed at the end of the intervention period.

[c] Difference between the time series modeled value in the absence of chlorhexidine bathing and the observed model value at the end of the intervention period with the percentage change in parenthesis.

From Climo MW, Sepkowitz KA, Zuccotti G, et al. The effect of daily bathing with chlorhexidine on the acquisition of methicillin-resistant Staphylococcus aureus, vancomycin-resistant Enterococcus, and healthcare-associated bloodstream infections: Results of a quasi-experimental multicenter trial. Crit Care Med 2009;37:1862; with permission.

Skin at the surgical site should be free of oils, soilage, grease, or other debris before the antiseptic skin preparation.

Antiseptics should be applied as per the manufacturer's recommendations. The outer boundaries of the skin preparation should be considerably wider than the direct area of the incision site. This allows for maximum antiseptic effect in areas that may be contacted during the actual operation. More than one applicator may be necessary.

Most antiseptics require vigorous back and forth scrubbing of the solution into the skin for a specified time period. Maximum contact is essential to achieve the greatest bacterial kill.

If areas of potentially greater bacterial colonization are present within the skin preparation area (eg, wounds, pubis, colostomy site), prepare these last. Use a second applicator for areas of higher contamination.

Allow to completely dry as per manufacturer's recommendations. Some active ingredients do not become active until drying occurs. This is also particularly important when using products that contain alcohol, which is flammable. Do not allow antiseptics to pool on the prepared area, under or around the patient. In addition, antiseptics need to be dry before the use of drapes.

Hands-free applicators are the best method to apply an antiseptic solution. Do not touch the prepared area after antiseptic has been applied. This reduces risk of contamination.

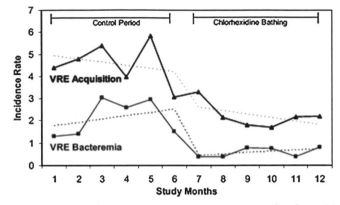

Fig. 2. Reduction in the rate of vancomycin-resistant *Enterococcus* (VRE) acquisition and VRE bacteremia associated with chlorhexidine bathing. Comparison of rate of the acquisition of VRE (▲) with the rate of incident VRE bacteremia (■). The dotted line represents the modeled trend based on time series analysis. During the baseline period (study months 1–6), all patients admitted to study units received regular bathing and during the intervention period (study months 7–12), all patients admitted to the study units received daily bathing with chlorhexidine. The rate of acquisition of VRE is the number of new cases of VRE per 1000 eligible patient–days. The rate of incident VRE bacteremias is the number of new cases of incident VRE bacteremias per 1000 total patient–days. (*From* Climo MW, Sepkowitz KA, Zuccotti G, et al. The effect of daily bathing with chlorhexidine on the acquisition of methicillin-resistant *Staphylococcus aureus*, vancomycin-resistant *Enterococcus*, and healthcare-associated bloodstream infections: Results of a quasi-experimental multicenter trial. Crit Care Med 2009;37:1858–65; with permission.)

Do not rinse or wipe the antiseptic solution off the skin. This is particularly important if CHG is used, since it provides long-term residual effect.

If necessary, additional antiseptic may be applied as long as the first application is allowed to dry. Remember that antiseptics such as CHG have cumulative effects after second applications. This is the intent when patients have preoperative antiseptic showers followed by preoperative skin preparation.

SUMMARY

The latest scientific information advances the knowledge of both methodology and type of antiseptic that should be used in most surgeries performed in the United States. The information contained here provides credible evidence that medical institutions should strongly consider revisions to their protocols that address skin antisepsis for their surgical patients. Preoperative showers for patients undergoing elective surgery should be implemented as part of a standard infection control program, with clear instructions to apply the solution in cloth form at both evening and morning before operation. Solution should not be rinsed off to assure high levels of CHG concentration. The operative scrub should be done in a vigorous back-and-forth manner to better achieve antiseptic–bacterial membrane contact of organisms in deeper layers of the skin. Finally, for patients in critical care areas, decontamination protocols should be instituted on a daily basis particularly aimed at reducing the risk of acquiring multidrug resistant organisms.

REFERENCES

1. Healthcare Infection Control Practices Advisory Committee, Centers for Disease Control and Prevention. Guideline for hand hygiene in healthcare settings. MMWR Morb Mortal Wkly Rep 2002;51(RR–16):1–56.
2. Denton GW. Chlorhexidine. In: Block SS, editor. Disinfection, sterilization, and preservation. 5th edition. Philadelphia: Lippincott Williams & Wilkens; 2001. p. 321–36.
3. Aly R, Malbach HI. Comparative antibacterial efficacy of a 2-minute surgical scrub with chlorhexidine gluconate, povidone-iodine, and chloroxylenol sponge brushes. Am J Infect Control 1988;16:173–7.
4. Peterson AF, Rosenberg A, Alatary SD. Comparison evaluation of surgical scrub preparations. Surg Gynecol Obstet 1978;146:63–5.
5. Hospital Infection Control Practices Advisory Committee, Centers for Disease Control and Prevention. Guideline for prevention of surgical site infection, 1999. Available at: http://www.cdc.gov/ncidod/dhqp/pdf/guidelines/SSI.pdf. Accessed February 23, 2010.
6. Garibaldi RA. Prevention of intraoperative wound contamination with chlorhexidine shower and scrub. J Hosp Infect 1988;11(Supp B):5–9.
7. Paulson DS. Efficacy evaluation of a 4% chlorhexidine gluconate as a full-body shower wash. Am J Infect Control 1993;21:205–9.
8. Hayek LJ, Emerson JM, Gardner AM. A placebo-controlled trial of the effect of two preoperative baths or showers with chlorhexidine detergent on postoperative wound infection rates. J Hosp Infect 1987;10(2):165–72.
9. Kaiser AB, Kernodle DA, Barg NL, et al. Influence of preoperative showers on staphylococcal skin colonization: a comparative trial of antiseptic skin cleansers. Ann Thorac Surg 1988;45:35–8.
10. Anderson DJ, Kaye KS, Classen D, et al. Strategies to prevent surgical site infections in acute care hospitals. SHEA/IDSA practice recommendation. Infect Control Hosp Epidemiol 2008;29:551–61.
11. Webster J, Osborne S. Preoperative bathing or showering with skin antiseptics to prevent surgical site infection. Cochrane Database Syst Rev 2009;3:1–34.
12. Perioperative standards and recommended practices, 2010 edition. Denver (Colorado): Association of periOperative Registered Nurses; 2010.
13. Edmiston CE, Krepel CJ, Seabrook GR, et al. Preoperative shower revisited: can high topical antiseptic levels be achieved on the skin surface before surgical admission. J Am Coll Surg 2008;207:233–9.
14. Bleadsdale SC, Trick WE, Gonzalez IM, et al. Effectiveness of chlorhexidine bathing to reduce catheter-associated bloodstream infections in medical intensive care unit patients. Arch Intern Med 2007;167:2073–9.
15. Karpanen TJ, Worthington T, Conway BR, et al. Penetration of chlorhexidine into human skin. Antimicrob Agents Chemother 2008;52:3633–6.
16. Byrne DJ, Napier A, Cuschieri A. The value of whole body disinfection in the prevention of post-operative wound infection in clean and potentially contaminated surgery. A prospective, randomized, double blind, placebo-controlled trial. Surg Res Comm 1992;12:43–52.
17. Earnshaw JJ, Berbridge DC, Slack RC, et al. Do preoperative chlorhexidine baths reduce the risk of infection after vascular reconstruction? Eur J Vasc Surg 1989;3(4):323–6.
18. Randall PE, Ganguli L, Marcuson RW. Wound infection following vasectomy. Br J Urol 1983;55(5):564–7.

19. Rotter ML, Larsen SO, Cooke EM, et al. A comparison of the effects of preoperative whole-body bathing with detergent alone and with detergent containing chlorhexidine gluconate on the frequency of wound infections after clean surgery. The European Working Party on Control of Hospital Infections. J Hosp Infect 1988;11(4):310–20.

20. Veiga DF, Damasceno CA, Veiga-Filho J, et al. Randomized controlled trial of the effectiveness of chlorhexidine showers before elective plastic surgery procedures. Infect Control Hosp Epidemiol 2009;30(1):77–9.

21. Wihlborg O. The effect of washing with chlorhexidine soap on wound infection rate in general surgery. A controlled clinical study. Ann Chir Gynaecol 1987; 76(5):263–5.

22. Maki DG, Ringer M, Alvarado CJ. Prospective, randomized trial of povidone–iodine, alcohol, and chlorhexidine for prevention of infection of infection associated with central venous and arterial catheters. Lancet 1991;338: 339–43.

23. Chaiyakunapruk N, Venestra DL, Lipsky BA, et al. Chlorhexidine compared with povidone–iodine solution for vascular catheter-site care: a meta-analysis. Ann Intern Med 2002;136:792–801.

24. Grabsch EA, Mitchell DJ, Hooper J, et al. In use-efficacy of a chlorhexidine in alcohol surgical rub: a comparative study. ANZ J Surg 2004;74:769–72.

25. Garcia R. A review of the possible role of oral and dental colonization on the occurrence of health care-associated pneumonia: underappreciated risk and a call for interventions. Am J Infect Control 2005;33:527–41.

26. Hibbard JS, Mulberry GK, Brady AR. A clinical study comparing the skin antisepsis and safety of chloraprep, 70% isopropyl alcohol, and 2% aqueous chlorhexidine. J Infus Nurs 2002;25:244–9.

27. Edwards P, Lipp A, Holmes A. Preoperative skin antiseptics for preventing surgical wound infections after clean surgery. Cochrane Database Syst Rev 2004;3:CD003949.

28. Berry A, Watt B, Goldacre M, et al. A comparison of the use of povidone–iodine and chlorhexidine in the prophylaxis. J Hosp Infect 1982;3:55–63.

29. Ellenhorn JD, Smith DD, Schwarz RE, et al. Paint-only is equivalent to scrub-and-paint in preoperative preparation of abdominal surgery sites. J Am Coll Surg 2005;201:737–41.

30. Darouiche RO, Wall MJ Jr, Itani KMF, et al. Chlorhexidine–alcohol versus povidone–iodine for surgical-site antisepsis. N Engl J med 2010;302.10–20.

31. Mannien J, Wille JC, Snoeren RL, et al. Impact of postdischarge surveillance on surgical site infection rates for several surgical procedures: results from the nosocomial surveillance network in The Netherlands. Infect Control Hosp Epidemiol 2006;27:809–16.

32. Wenzel RP. Minimizing surgical site infections. N Engl J med 2010;362:75–7.

33. Vernon MO, Hayden MK, Trick WE, et al. Chlorhexidine gluconate to cleanse patients in a medical intensive care unit. Arch Intern Med 2006;166:306–12.

34. Climo MW, Sepkowitz KA, Zuccotti G, et al. The effect of daily bathing with chlorhexidine on the acquisition of methicillin-resistant *Staphylococcus aureus*, vancomycin-resistant *Enterococcus*, and healthcare-associated bloodstream infections: results of a quasi-experimental multicenter trial. Crit Care Med 2009; 37:1858–65.

35. Popovich KJ, Hota B, Hayes R, et al. Effectiveness of routine patient cleansing with chlorhexidine gluconate for infection prevention in the medical intensive care unit. Infect Control Hosp Epidemiol 2009;30:959–63.

36. Holder C, Zellinger M. Daily bathing with chlorhexidine in the ICU to prevent central line-associated bloodstream infections. J Clin Outcomes Manag 2009; 16:509–13.

37. Batra R, Cooper BS, Whiteley C, et al. Efficacy and limitation of a chlorhexidine-based decolonization strategy in preventing transmission of methicillin-resistant *Staphylococcus aureus* in an intensive care unit. Clin Infect Dis 2010;50:210–7.

38. Association of Surgical Technologists. Recommended standards of practice for skin prep of the surgical patient October 2008. Available at: http://www.ast.org/pdf/Standards_of_Practice/RSOP_Skin_Prep.pdf. Accessed June 6, 2010.

39. Carrico R. 7 steps to better prepping. Available at: http://www.outpatientsurgery.net/guides/infection-control/2009/7-teps-to-better-prepping&pg=2. Accessed July 3, 2010.

Improving the Process of Supplying Instruments to the Operating Room Using the Lean Rapid Cycle Improvement Process

Kathi Mullaney, BSN, MPH, CIC

KEYWORDS
- Quality improvement • Lean • Operating room
- Central sterile services • Surgical instruments

Concepts of quality improvement are not new to the health care environment, and in fact these concepts are being used more frequently to improve and enhance health care delivery in all areas of the health care milieu from medical intensive care units, the operating room, social services, and environmental services. One quality improvement process that is gaining in popularity is the lean method. In the operating room, author and colleagues identified that there was an increase in surgical cases being delayed or cancelled. They used the lean process to get to the root of the problem and improve the processes the author and colleagues had been using for supplying the operating room with the sterile instruments used for surgical procedures on a daily basis.

LEAN PRINCIPLES

Lean principles have been used effectively in manufacturing companies for decades. The concept of lean is commonly associated with Japanese manufacturing, specifically the Toyota Production System based on W. Edwards Deming. Lean thinking is based on managers focusing on improving the production process and building quality into the product on the first try. Lean means using less to do more. It is a systematic approach for identifying and eliminating waste through continuous improvement. Lean improves processes and outcomes, reduces cost, reduces cycle times and ultimately increases

Department of Infection Control, Metropolitan Hospital, 1901 First Avenue, New York, NY 10029, USA
E-mail address: Kathi.mullaney@nychhc.org

Perioperative Nursing Clinics 5 (2010) 479–487
doi:10.1016/j.cpen.2010.09.001
1556-7931/10/$ – see front matter © 2010 Elsevier Inc. All rights reserved.

patient and staff satisfaction. The goal of lean is to deliver higher quality patient services in the most efficient effective and responsive manner possible.

In their 1996 book *Lean Thinking,* James Womack and Daniel Jones presented lean as consisting of set of five basic principles. They described the characteristics of a lean organization as having the following ideals:

Specify value—identifying the value of their product from the standpoint of the end customer. In health care the end customer is the patient. The concept is that the value is most meaningful when it meets the patient's needs at a specific price at a specific time. An example would be canceling a case due to lack of instruments, incomplete preoperative workup, or improper health insurance validation. Was the patient's time valued?

Value stream—identify all steps that provide value for the patient for each product family and eliminating every step and every action and every practice that does not create value.

Flow—make the value-creating steps occur in a tight and integrated sequence so the product or process for patient care will flow smoothly through the patient procedure or care. This step requires a fundamental change in the usual way of thinking in the traditional health care system. The phrase "we have been doing it this way for the last…." is no longer the standard. One needs to think out of the box to improve flow.

Pull value—as flow is introduced, allow the patients to pull value from their next upstream activity. The institution must make the commitment to provide patients with services that contribute to the quality of their care and enhance their visits. The visit should have value for the patients. The patient will be given relevant postoperative teaching, prescriptions, or medications, and their first postoperative follow-up appointment will be made before they are discharged.

Pursue perfection—as these steps lead to greater transparency, enabling managers and teams to eliminate further waste. Pursuing perfection is through continuous improvement. There is no end to the process of reducing effort, time, space, cost, and mistakes when providing patient care. The patient is the customer, and one must provide a perfect product to ensure their safety.[1]

LEAN THINKING IN THE HEALTH CARE ENVIRONMENT

Introducing lean thinking requires buy in from the entire organization or health care system. It cannot be successful if only middle managers or frontline staff drive the momentum. It must be led by those at the very top of the organization. Success depends on a strong commitment and inspiring leadership from senior staff for this very challenging effort. The chief executive officer (CEO) must be a vocal, visible champion of Lean management, create an environment where it is permissible to fail, set previously unheard of goals, and encourage leaps of faith. Going lean must be an integral part of the senior staff vision. The vision will provide the health care workers a guide to make the right choices.

Traditional culture in the organization must evolve into a new culture. Examples of traditional culture versus lean culture may include:

Functioning in silos versus interdisciplinary teams
Blame people versus root cause analysis
Volume lowers cost versus removing waste lowers cost.

Health care workers traditionally see their work as valuable and do not see patients as customers. However, the added dimension of lean is recognizing and critically changing the amount of time wasted trying to provide care to patients (customers). In the operating room, this can be seen in delayed operating room start times. Is it the culture to start 15 minutes late; does the transporter complete multiple tasks before delivering the patient thus delaying start time, or does one only have one set of instruments for a very active service, because there always has been only one set, again delaying start time of the case?

Lean provides a framework to review the process of delivering valuable health care to patients. Primary processes serve the external customers, the patient and family. Internal processes serve the internal customers such as the staff, insurers, government, and payers. Value must be focused on creating processes that define the primary customer, the patient. The process must be valuable, capable, available, adequately flexible, and linked by continuous flow to prevent waste.[2]

WASTES

The basic concept of the lean method focuses on eliminating seven wastes:

Inventory—overstocked, obsolete or incorrect items thus money is wasted
Motion—walking waste stems from poor design or lack of optimal conditions
Transportation—moving patients, tests, materials, or information around
Over processing—multiple billing
Defects—unlabelled specimens, incomplete medical records
Waiting—patients waiting to be seen, to be admitted, or to complete a test
Underutilizing staff—failure to incorporate the end user staff in the decision-making process, hiring consultants to solve internal problems.

The plan-do-study-act (PDSA) cycle is the lean working structure—the system for executing Kaizen. The term Kaizen is derived from two Japanese characters; kai, measuring change and zen meaning continuous improvement. Eliminating waste in the value stream is the goal of Kaizen.[3] Lean elevates PDSA to a level of immediate accomplishments. However, sustaining the accomplishments requires continuous use of the PDSA cycle.

PLAN-DO-STUDY-ACT CYCLE

The PDSA cycle (**Fig. 1**) is a four-step model for performing change. Just as a circle has no end, the PDSA cycle should be repeated again and again for continuous improvement.

Plan-do-study-act should be used

As a model for continuous improvement
When starting a new improvement project
When developing a new or improved design of a process, product, or service
When defining a repetitive work process
When planning data collection and analysis to verify and prioritize problems or root causes
When implementing any change.

The plan-do-study-act process can be described as:

Plan. Recognize an opportunity and plan a change.
Do. Test the change. Carry out a small-scale study.
Study. Review the test, analyze the results, and identify what has been learned.

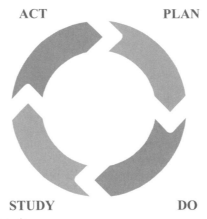

Fig. 1. Plan-do-study-act cycle.

Act. Take action based on what has been learned in the study step. If the change did not work, go through the cycle again with a different plan. If success was achieved, incorporate what has been learned from the test into wider changes. Use what has been learned to plan new improvements, beginning the cycle again.[3]

IMPLEMENTING A LEAN PROJECT

The first step in lean is to define the value stream. The organization needs to distinguish value-added and nonvalue-added steps to ultimately create flow and eliminate waste. The leaders in the organization identify, by product family, the value of the processes in the designated departments. The product family could be the ambulatory services, the operating room, or the emergency department just to name a few. The senior management team and the executive sponsor provide guidance on the processes to be improved to achieve the hospital goals of patient safety, patient satisfaction, employee satisfaction, and fiscal responsibility.

A 4- to 5 day rapid improvement event (RIE) is conducted with a select group of front-line staff, managers, physicians, and senior staff to analyze the identified problem. The team must continually ask why until the root cause of the problem is determined.

The lean methodology employs A3 thinking during the RIE. The A3 report is a tool that Toyota uses to propose solutions to problems, give status reports on ongoing projects, and report results of information-gathering activities. The A3 problem-solving method is a way to look with fresh eyes at a specific problem identified in an organized manner. It is a tool with a structured approach that forces the user to thoroughly define and understand the issue, address it with improvement, and manage the corrections. An A3:

Is logic condensed on an 11 × 17 inch sheet of paper
Is a story without a storyteller
Structures the activities of the RIE
Shares knowledge
Builds quality.

The structure of the A3 depends on the project; however, the report or tool contains seven main elements that follow one another in a logical and organized sequence: background, current situation and problem, goals and targets, root cause analysis, action items and proposed implementation plan, verification measures, and follow-up. The steps included in the A3 tool used for my example include: reason for action, initial state, target state, gap analysis, solution approach, rapid experiment, completion plan, confirmed state, and lessons learned.[4–7]

APPLYING LEAN THINKING IN THE OPERATING ROOM

In the spring of 2009, an RIE was convened to improve the process of supplying central sterile instruments to the operating room. The members of the team included the administrator for central sterile supply (CSS), the central sterile manager, the operating room head nurse, chief of the dental service, the infection control manager, a central sterile technician, and the psychiatry outpatient manager, who was the team leader. The director of CSS was the process owner, and the chief of surgery was the executive sponsor.

Reason For Action

Perioperative services perform around 7000 surgical procedures annually, approximately 20 surgical cases per day. Approximately 10% of the cases each year, one to two cases each day, are delayed or cancelled because of missing, mislabeled or defective CSS instruments. Delays have the potential of negatively impacting patient safety and operating room efficiency.

Initial State

The team brainstormed and completed a waste walk (gemba walk). During this exercise, the team visited CSS, talked to the staff, and observed work practices. They found:

There are operating room cancellations and delays caused by missing, mislabeled, or defective CSS instruments.

CSS is processing 30 to 40 trays daily for 20 operating room cases because of trays with missing, mislabeled, defective, or incorrect instruments.

Instruments are flashed in the operating room by the operating room nurses and technicians.

Computerized database has generalized and incomplete data/illustrations and is not being optimally used in CSS and the operating room.

Target State

The team completed the metric using the data collected during the waste walk. The team identified the target state that would be implemented and demonstrated measures of success (**Table 1**). How can one ensure a waste free process?

No cancellations or delays due to missing, mislabeled, or defective CSS instruments
All instruments and trays will be processed in CSS exclusively

Table 1 Target state		
Metric	**Baseline**	**Target**
CSS Travel Time to Replace Broken or Missing Instruments	60ft (limited access)	5ft (full access)
Rate of Tray Processing per OR Cases Daily	1.5	1.0
Flashes per Month (%)	7	0
Number of Cases Canceled per Day	2	0

Abbreviation: OR, operating room.

Table 2 Gap analysis	
Gap	**Root Cause**
Central sterile supply (CSS) staff are not able to prioritize processing of trays	CSS staff do not have correlated information between operating room schedule and related trays
Multipart instruments are missing parts or have malfunctioning mechanisms Instruments are not functioning properly	Limited training of CSS and operating room staff in processing multipart instruments and identification of instrument malfunctions
Damaged and missing instruments are not replaced in a timely manner	Standard work not established for identifying such instruments.

Create standard work for identifying and replacing missing and damaged instruments
Update computerized database to include specific data/illustrations.

Gap Analysis

This provides a framework of changes that must be implemented to achieve the target state. The team members analyze the information and observations of the waste walk and provide the root causes. What is keeping the team from achieving the target state? How does one close the gaps and get to the root cause of the problem? Using the five whys is a very effective tool that forces the team to drill down to the real causes of the problem and the effects. **Table 2** outlines the results of the gap analysis.

Solution Approach

This exercise crystallizes the gap analysis. The team can implement the appropriate fix during the RIE. This is the working session of the RIE. During this exercise the team implements solutions or performs rapid experiments. This is accomplished by the team collaborating with consultants from within the facility such as information technology (IT) or facilities management. The consultants provide the expertise needed to operationalize the rapid experiments. **Table 3** outlines the solution approach process.

Table 3 Solution approach	
If One	**Then One**
Has correct information regarding the operating room schedule and trays needed	Can prioritize sterilization process to accommodate operating room case needs
Trains central sterile supply (CSS) and operating room staff to identify multipart and nonfunctioning instruments	Minimizes cannibalization of other sterile trays during operating room procedures
Standardizes workflow including the increased availability of and training in the terminal for the CSS and operating room staff	Will uniformly incorporate the terminal system to efficiently identify and track instrumentation
Establish par levels and standard work for identifying damaged and missing instruments	One can maintain the integrity of the trays
Has daily huddles in the operating room	Will increase communication between CSS staff and the OR staff

Table 4 Rapid experiment				
Experiments	**Baseline**	**Expected Outcome**	**Actual Outcome**	**Comments**
Affix bar codes on the instrument trays with the count sheets	84%	100%	92%	For hard trays or frequently used trays
Create a shared drive for preference card list	-	100%	80%	All users have not been added
Create standard work for processing instruments	-	100%	50%	The manager is working with the staff to establish standard work for all stations
Place peg board at the work station to reduce distance traveled	-	100%	100%	Purchased and installed within 60 days of rapid improvement event

Rapid Experiment

The established solutions are operationalized during this exercise with the cooperation of the CSS staff. The rapid experiments are performed in real time. This provides the team and the staff with a sense of reality and completion, an objective measurement of the task and knowledge that the solutions can be implemented. **Table 4** outlines the process of the rapid experiment.

Completion Plan

Tasks not completed during the RIE are assigned a timeframe for completion. **Table 5** outlines the process and documentation where staff commits to completion dates that are reported at the 120-day report.

Confirmed State

Table 6 provides a visual measurement of the successes and accomplishments at the 120 day mark.
   Lessons learned include:

   Improved communication between the CSS and OR staff
   Improved accuracy of the OR trays
   Decreased flashing
   Increased efficiency of CSS staff.

Table 5 Completion plan		
What	**Who**	**When**
Establish par Levels for Instrumentation	Nursing	6/1/09
Complete standard work for processing instruments	Central sterile	4/15/09
Update surgeon preference list	Nursing	On-going
Install 2 additional terminals	Administration	4/17/09
Schedule terminal training for central sterile supply and operating room staff	Administration	4/9/09

Table 6 Confirmed state							
Metrics	Start	Final Rapid Improvement Event	30 Days May	60 Days June	90 Days July	120 Days August	Target
Central Sterile Supply Travel Time to Replace Broken or Missing Instruments	60 ft	60 ft	60 ft	5 ft	5 ft	5 ft	5 ft
Flashes per Month (Excluding Contaminated Instruments) (%)	7	7	6	5	6	4	0
Count Sheets Matching Terminal (%)	49	49	59	90	90	90	100
Number of Cases Canceled per Day	2	2	0	0	0	0	0

Out Brief

Everyone is invited to the out brief in the auditorium. Most importantly, the audience must include the customers of the event. Each member of the team participates in the presentation of the RIE. The audience is invited to ask questions and provide comments and praise. Executive leadership has a major presence at the presentation.

IS THAT ALL THERE IS?

The out brief is not the end rather the beginning of implementing the improvements on a daily basis. It is critical that leadership continues to support the staff during the

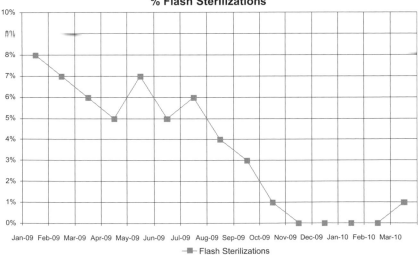

Fig. 2. Monthly rate of flash sterilization.

change, reinforce the new common vision, and coach the staff to sustain the change. Follow-up for this project was established through daily huddles, 30-, 60-, 90-, and 120-day updates. Eventually support begins to grow; staff develops pride, and a culture of change emerges. The lean framework encourages the process of continuous improvement demonstrated by the plan-do-study-act cycle. There continues to be a corporate commitment to lean, with the operating room identified as a value stream.

Success

Fig. 2 illustrates an example of sustained improvement. During the RIE, flash sterilization was addressed as a problem because of the identified instrument issues. After the RIE, CSS and the operating room head nurse huddled daily to ensure the operating room had the necessary instruments with good outcomes. They continue to huddle at least once per week. Flashing is reduced dramatically due to the outcomes of the RIE.

Using the lean process has resulted in a change in culture for the author's operating room, virtually eliminating delays caused by the lack of supply of sterile surgical instruments for the daily surgical procedures. Operating room efficiency has increased; patient safety has improved, and staff members in CSS and the OR continue to improve collaboration and communication.

REFERENCES

1. Womack J, Jones DT. Lean thinking. New York: Simon & Schuster; 1996.
2. Institute For Healthcare Improvement (IHI) White Paper. Going lean in healthcare. Cambridge (UK): IHI; 2005.
3. Tague N. The quality toolbox. Milwaukee (WI): ASQ Quality Press; 2004.
4. Consulting Simpler. Simpler design system. Available at: www.simpler.com. Accessed August, 2010.
5. Hagood C. Lean at work from factory floor to operating room. Available at: www. isixsigma. Accessed August 23, 2010.
6. Kimsey D. Lean methodology in health care. AORN J 2010;92(1):53–60.
7. Manos A, Salter M, Alukal G. Make healthcare lean. Qual Prog 2006;39(7):24–30.

Collaboration Among Central Sterile Processing, Surgical Services, and Infection Prevention and Control Finds Solutions of Increased Positive Biologic Cultures During Flash Sterilization in the Operating Room

Mary Ann Magerl, RN, MA, CIC[a],*, Mary Olivera, MS, CRCST, CHL, FCS[b]

KEYWORDS

- Biologic testing • Sterilizers • Flash sterilization
- Biologic failures of sterilization • Performance improvement

Black holes are concentrated areas of mass that are so immense that the considerable force of gravity does not allow anything within a certain area around it from passing through. Black holes have been given their names because light inside this event horizon can never be seen by mankind or any outside observer. Black holes are known to exist not because one can see them but because of the effect they have on the space around them. In health care institutions, 2 areas are generally viewed as alien territory or as unknown, and the author has likened them to and identified them as black holes. One is the central sterile processing (CSP) and the other is the operating room (OR). Most health care workers know that the CSP is where cleaning and reprocessing of surgical instruments take place and that the OR is where patients undergo surgery, but these workers have limited knowledge about the daily and ongoing

[a] Department of Infection Prevention and Control, Westchester Medical Center, Macy Pavilion, 2nd floor SW 246, Room 2080, Valhalla, NY 10595, USA
[b] Case Medical, Inc, 19 Empire Boulevard, South Hackensack, NJ 07606, USA
* Corresponding author.
E-mail address: mamicp@aol.com

Perioperative Nursing Clinics 5 (2010) 489–500
doi:10.1016/j.cpen.2010.07.002
1556-7931/10/$ – see front matter © 2010 Elsevier Inc. All rights reserved.

workings and functioning of these areas; hence these areas are viewed as 2 black holes. The CSP and OR are 2 areas of high specialization that are actually interwoven in their functional procedures relative to positive outcomes in patients who need surgical interventions.

The opportunity to collaborate on a patient safety issue brought these 2 groups together to focus on the problem and helped develop a well-functioning team that was then able to address many other identified issues. This article discusses how this group was able to develop, become a team, collaborate, and use several different tools to find the cause and implement a solution for the increased presence of positive biologic cultures found during flash sterilization.

Collaboration is the process by which 2 or more groups work together on an intersection of common goals that are relative in nature by sharing knowledge, learning, and building consensus. Collaboration is the central problem in any collective undertaking and is based on the premise that professionals want to work together to realize positive outcomes.[1] Most collaboration requires leadership, although the form of leadership can be social within a decentralized and equalitarian milieu as is found in health care settings. There are many challenges associated with collaboration; probably the one that receives the least amount of attention is the overuse of the language and therefore the misinterpretation of concepts. The complexity of the work in health care requires that everyone work together on a variety of issues. A working definition of collaboration is joining together to make possible something that cannot be accomplished alone. Collaboration requires the partnership and the commitment of all members working toward a common goal to succeed. High-performance teams have a clear understanding of the goal to be achieved and a belief that the goal is worthwhile or that the result is important. Having a clear goal permits the team to understand clearly that it will achieve its goal. This highly effective team was asked to resolve the identified problem, establish an innovation, and complete a well-defined plan.

At each group meeting, roles and accountabilities were clarified, lines of communication were established, plans for monitoring performance and providing feedback were established, and when challengers were identified, factual data were used and experts were requested to join the team to address perceived issues following the principles of collaborative justice.[2] The members of the team included staff from the surgical services, CSP, infection prevention and control (IC), and administration. Team members had 3 common features: essential skills and abilities to conduct the specific work, a strong desire to contribute, and the capacity to collaborate effectively.

THE PROBLEM

An increase in the number of failed biologic tests was identified in the main OR of an urban medical center. In spite of many efforts to resolve the problem, the number of test failures continued to increase. To better understand the problem, a performance improvement team (PIT) was developed. The team was integrated with members of the surgical services, CSP, IC, hospital information systems, and microbiology personnel. A member of the hospital information system was selected because all orders for the microbiology laboratory were sent electronically using a designed pathway. The microbiology department was also included because the technicians are responsible for incubating and certifying the results of the biologic tests on the sterilizers. A risk assessment was completed in conjunction with a fishbone diagram (**Fig. 1**). All members of the team contributed and provided input to categorize the cause of the problem as it linked through the process. Using the plan, do, check, and act performance improvement methodology, a root-cause analysis was

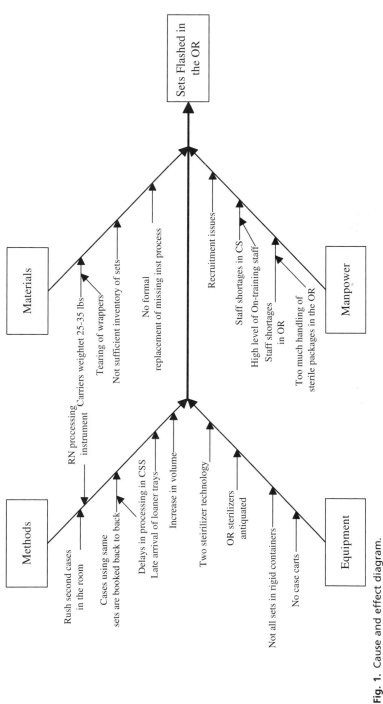

Fig. 1. Cause and effect diagram.

performed. This analysis was used to explore and display the possible causes of the problem and give the PIT the tools to begin making variations in the process (**Box 1**).

STERILIZATION PRACTICE STANDARDS

Practice, guidelines and standards for reprocessing and sterilizing instruments and supplies that are used during surgical procedures, including flash sterilization, are available. The Joint Commission (TJC) requires that departments/services performing decontamination and sterilization activities have written policies and procedures (P&Ps) related to these activities.

These P&Ps must be consistent or standardized throughout the organization. The monitoring of the sterilization process and its documentation must also be standardized in addition to having a well-defined structure outlining the responsibility for monitoring sterilizer performance. The TJC has also updated the IC standard and its elements of performance (EP). The new rationale for the standards that they provided are intended to clarify requirements to reduce the risks associated with medical equipment, devices, and supplies. In 2010, the National Patient Safety Goals were released for ambulatory care, critical access hospital, office-based surgery, and so on. The IC standard IC.02.02.01 and its EP 1 and EP 2 for ambulatory care, critical care access hospitals, office-based surgery, and so on were effective immediately. There has been noted confusion in the field about the applicability of Standard IC.02.02.01. Because EP 1 refers to cleaning and disinfection, it applies to lower-risk processes. However, EP 2 refers to sterilization and consequently applies to higher-risk processes, which include intermediate- and high-level disinfection.

The TJC survey process continues to be focused on

- Orientation, training, and competency of the health care workers who process medical equipment, devices, and supplies
- Levels of staffing and supervision of the health care workers who process medical equipment, devices, and supplies
- Standardization of the process regardless of whether it is centralized or decentralized

---

Box 1
Sidebar

Tools used

Plan, Do, Check, and Act

Plan, do, check, and act is based on the scientific method developed in 1620 from the work of Francis Bacon Novum Organum. This method permits one to monitor the rate of improvement and has permitted for major jumps. This tool is used with sizable projects that would require numerous people to contribute their time. Thus, it shows managers the larger picture and enables breakthrough improvements to justify the effort expended.

Fishbone mapping

Sometimes called a herringbone map, a fishbone map is a type of graphic organizer that is used to explore the many aspects or effects of a complex topic. The process of creating a fishbone diagram helps to focus on the topic, requires the user to review what was already known to organize that knowledge, and helps the team to monitor its comprehension of the problem. This diagram helps to point out the area where the team must investigate more.

- Ongoing quality monitoring
- Observation against the manufacturer's guidelines and the organization's procedures.[3]

Documentation is another aspect of these standards of practice. Both the TJC and the Association for periOperative Registered Nurses (AORN) recommend that any item that has been flash sterilized should be recorded and traceable back to a sterilizer and a patient in the event of a biologic test failure. This documentation must be a standard practice, and in some organizations, computerized record keeping facilitates the task of monitoring the performance of the staff and the equipment. These recommended practices were developed by the AORN Recommended Practices Committee and have been approved by the AORN Board of Directors. The recommendations represent what is believed to be an optimal level of practice and provide guidance for sterilizing items that are to be used in the surgical environment.[4]

A major responsibility of the perioperative registered nurse is to minimize patient risk for surgical site infection (SSI). One measure for preventing SSI is to provide surgical items that are free of contamination at the time of use. Sterilization provides the highest level of assurance that surgical items are free of viable microbes.

Recommendations for flash sterilization are as follows:

- Use of flash sterilization should be kept to a minimum. Flash sterilization should be used only in selected clinical situations and in a controlled manner. Flash sterilization may be associated with an increased risk of infection to patients because of the pressure on personnel to eliminate one or more steps in the cleaning and sterilization process.
- Proper decontamination is essential in removing bioburden and preparing an item for sterilization by any method. Flash sterilization should be performed only if all of the following conditions are met:
  The device manufacturer's written instructions on the cycle type, exposure times, temperature settings, and drying times are available and followed.
  Items are disassembled and thoroughly cleaned with detergent and water to remove soil, blood, body fats, and other substances.
  Lumens are brushed and flushed under water with a cleaning solution and rinsed thoroughly.
  Items are placed in a closed sterilization container or tray validated for flash sterilization, in a manner that allows steam to contact all instrument surfaces.
  Measures are taken to prevent contamination during transfer to the sterile field.
  Flash sterilized items are to be used immediately and not stored for later use.
- Packaging and wrapping should not be used in flash sterilization cycles unless the sterilizer is specifically designed and labeled for this use.
- Sterilizer manufacturer's written directions should be followed and reconciled with the packaging manufacturer's instructions for sterilization.
  Process challenge devices should be used with routine process monitoring devices. Process challenge and process monitoring devices provide information to demonstrate that conditions for sterilization have been met.
  Each sterilization cycle should be monitored to verify that parameters required for sterilization have been met.
  The sterilizer operator should use physical monitoring devices to verify cycle parameters for each load. Physical monitoring devices can indicate immediate sterilizer failure. Physical monitors record cycle parameters.

Biologic indicators (BIs) and chemical indicators should be used to monitor sterilizer efficacy and assess compliance of monitoring standards established for gravity displacement and dynamic air removal sterilizer. Class 5 chemical integrating indicators should be used within each sterilizer container or tray.

Users should adhere to aseptic techniques for flash sterilized items during transport to the point of use. It is important that sterilization processing be performed in a clean environment and that flash sterilized devices be transferred to the point of use in a manner that prevents contamination.

Rigid sterilization containers designed and intended for flash sterilization cycles should be used.

Flash sterilization containers should be used, cleaned, and maintained according to the manufacture's written instructions. Containers should be opened, used immediately, and not stored for later use. Also, these containers should be differentiated from other types of containers.

Flash sterilization should not be used for implantable devices, except in cases of emergency when no other option is available. In an emergency, when flash sterilization of an implant is unavoidable, a rapid-action BI with a Class 5 chemical integrating indicator should be run with the load. The implant should be quarantined on the back table and should not be released until the rapid-action BI provides a negative result. If the implant is used before the final report of the BI is known and the BI later provides a positive result, the surgeon and the IC personnel should be notified as soon as the results are known. If the implant is not used, it has to be resterilized before use.

Documentation of cycle information and monitoring results should be maintained in a log (electronic or manual) to provide tracking of the flashed items to the individual patient. Documentation allows every load of sterilized items used on patients to be traced.

The records should include information such as the items processed, the patient receiving the items, the cycle parameters used, the date and time the cycle is run, the operator information, and the reason for flash sterilization.[4]

THE ASSOCIATION FOR THE ADVANCEMENT OF MEDICAL INSTRUMENTATION STANDARDS

The Association for the Advancement of Medical Instrumentation (AAMI) was founded in 1967. The association's mission is to assist in the development, evaluation, acquisition, use, and maintenance of medical devices and instrumentation. The AAMI is widely recognized as one of the principal voluntary standards organizations in the United States. The AAMI Recommended Practice Standard, American National Standards Institute (ANSI)/AAMI ST79:2006, is a comprehensive guide to steam sterilization and sterility assurance in health care facilities. The following are the recommended practices as it relates to flash sterilization:

- A flash sterilization cycle is one that has been designed to meet the following criteria:

  The cycle is preprogrammed to a specific time-temperature setting established by the manufacturer based on the type of sterilizer control and selected by the user based on the configuration of the load.

  The items to be processed are usually unwrapped, although a single wrapper may be used in certain circumstances, that is, if the sterilizer or packaging manufacture's instructions permit.

Because drying time is not usually part of a preprogrammed flash cycle, the items processed are assumed to be wet at the conclusion of the cycle.

The processed items must be transferred immediately, using aseptic technique, from the sterilizer to the actual point of use, usually the sterile field in an ongoing surgical procedure. There is no storage or shelf life for flash sterilized items.

- It is essential for health care personnel to properly carry out the complete multi-step process when flash sterilization is used.
- Several concerns stimulated the development of guidelines for flash sterilization:

The Committee was aware of inadequate cleaning and other lapses in decontamination procedures before flash sterilization. Reduction of bioburden and removal of gross soil are essential steps in preparing an item for sterilization by any method.

Documentation of the flash sterilization process is necessary and should be consistent with the requirements applicable to and the practices used in documenting the routine processing of wrapped loads.

Items that are flash sterilized should be transported to the point of use in such a way that the potential for contamination is minimized.

- Flash sterilization of instruments should be considered only if all of the following conditions are met:

Work practices ensure proper cleaning and decontamination, inspection, and arrangement of instruments into the recommended sterilizing trays or other containment devices before sterilization.

The physical layout of the department or work area ensures direct delivery of sterilized items to the point of use.

Procedures are developed, followed, and audited to ensure aseptic handling and personnel safety during transfer of the sterilized items from the sterilizer to the point of use.

The item is needed for use immediately after flash sterilization.

- Implantable devices should not be flash sterilized.[5]

GUIDELINE FOR DISINFECTION AND STERILIZATION IN HEALTH CARE FACILITIES

The Guideline for Disinfection and Sterilization in Healthcare Facilities, 2008, is evidence-based recommendation on the preferred methods for cleaning, disinfection, and sterilization of patient-care medical devices. Beginning in October 2008, the Centers for Medicare and Medicaid Services do not reimburse facilities for care necessitated by certain avoidable errors, including SSIs in selected procedures.

Specific information related to the flash sterilization process in the guidelines are

- Do not flash sterilize implanted surgical devices unless doing so is unavoidable.
- Do not use flash sterilization for convenience, as an alternative to purchasing additional instrument sets, or to save time.
- When using flash sterilization, make sure the following parameters are met: (1) clean the item before placing it in the sterilizing container (which is cleared for use with flash sterilization by the US Food and Drug Administration) or tray, (2) prevent exogenous contamination of the item during transport from the sterilizer to the patient, and (3) monitor sterilizer function with mechanical, chemical, and biologic monitors.
- Do not use packaging materials and containers in flash sterilization cycles unless the sterilizer and the packaging materials or containers are designed for this use.
- When necessary, use flash sterilization for patient-care items that are used immediately (eg, to reprocess an inadvertently dropped instrument).

- When necessary, use flash sterilization for processing patient-care items that cannot be packaged, sterilized, and stored before use.[6]

FINDING THE ROOT CAUSE AND IMPLEMENTING CHANGE

The root-cause analysis helped the team to identify and categorize potential causes in an orderly manner and to define the problem. Some categories identified were

Method, machine, materials, manpower
Places, procedures, people, policies
Surroundings, supplies, systems, skills.

It should be remembered that when a problem occurs, it is usually a systems problem and has occurred on many levels and departments. During this process, one is able to identify the problem and put in a process to eliminate it. The first step for the process improvement team was to identify the problem: an increase in the number of positive biologic cultures in the flash sterilizer in the OR. The goal of the project was to reduce the number of sterilizer biologic test failures and that of the organization was to use a coordinated process to reduce the risks of endemic and epidemic infections in patients and staff as a result of sterilization process failures. The objective was also directed to improve the safety, efficacy, and efficiency of the sterilization process as well as the performance of the staff.

The team brainstormed the problem and carefully analyzed every step in the process. There were different causes that were found to be associated with the increase in the sterilization process failure. The first-level cause of the problem related to staff education because of a change in the product used to conduct biologic culture test, resulting in operator errors. In addition, different types of sterilizer recording devices were indirectly linked to the problem. Re-education was needed for the surgical services and microbiology staff to eliminate the problem. The documentation aspect of the process also needed revision because the hospital information system used to record the test information was not user friendly. As a result, the staff were using the wrong pathways, creating a problem for the laboratory technicians when they entered the test results. The laboratory staff also needed to understand the biologic test process to expedite the results and avoid delays in notifying sterilization process test failures.

To improve the process, the team identified that there was a need to implement intensive training to all staff. Continuing education sessions were held outlining the sterilization process, the sterilizer parameters to be expected in a completed cycle, and the biologic test procedure. Designated staff in the surgical services areas were trained and qualified to conduct the weekly biologic testing of the sterilizers, thereby decreasing the probability for operator's errors.

The microbiology laboratory technicians spent a few hours in sterile processing to learn about the sterilization process, the biologic tests, and their importance. This training helped the technicians to understand the urgency and the critical importance of the timing for obtaining the final negative biologic culture result.

The multidisciplinary group also standardized all record keeping in surgical service and central sterile areas. The sterilizer logbooks were designed to meet the requirements of the regulatory agencies and distributed to all surgical services for use. The computerized hospital information system screens were redesigned to require the same sterilization process test information throughout the surgical services and the sterile processing department. Individual log-in codes to the system were given to the staff for accountability purposes. The codes would easily identify the person conducting the test and entering the information. The new redesigned hospital

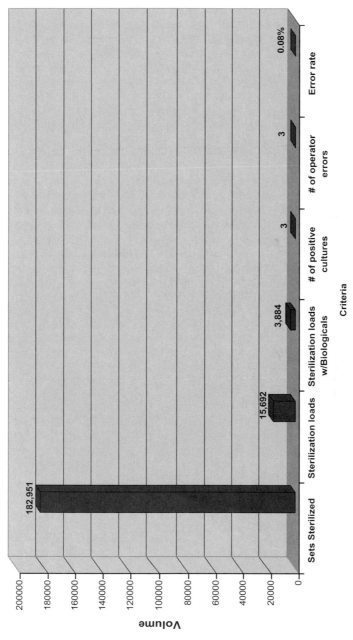

Fig. 2. Sterilization monitoring done by the central sterile processing.

information screens and the standardization of information facilitated the retrieval of biologic cultures test results because the microbiology laboratory was responsible for the incubation of the cultures.

Continued monitoring revealed that the error rate due to operator error decreased to less than 1% (0.08%) in the first 3 months of implementing the process improvement and decreased to 0% thereafter (**Fig. 2**). The continued monitoring of the efficiency and efficacy of the process was done by the IC team. A Report on Positive Test for Sterilizers form is completed and submitted to the hospital information system team listing the details and findings of the test failure, with an explanation of the corrective action taken. This form (Appendix 1) serves as a quality assurance tool, and, at the same time, underlines any deviation from the standard operating process. The data collected from these forms are shared with the departments for them to follow up on their progress. The IC team also conducts unscheduled visits to monitor compliance with practices.

A MULTIDISCIPLINARY EFFORT

Organizing a group by integrating different members of all the departments involved in the process served as a catalyst for success. Eliminating a problem can sometimes create another problem if all of the essential players are not included because causes that may lead to a problem might be left unresolved. A PIT can help to find the root cause of the problem and improve interdisciplinary communication and relationships.

The most important thing to remember about sterilization is that the standards are not different because of the setting. Regardless of the sterilization modality, the sterilizer type, the cycle selected, or the setting, the objective is the same. At the end of the cycle, a sterility assurance level (SAL) of 10^{-6} must be achieved for the device to be considered safe for use on a patient. Achieving this level requires that the sterilizer functions properly and that all related processes, such as cleaning and packaging, are done properly. In essence, achieving a sterility level of SAL 10^{-6} increases the probability of viable microorganisms remaining on a device after sterilization to be equal to or less than one in a million.[7]

All properly functioning sterilizers must be able to achieve an SAL of 10^{-6}. The ability to achieve this can be verified by periodic testing with a BI, specifically for the sterilization modality and cycle for which verification is desired. However, ensuring that a product is sterile for use in surgery means more than making sure that the sterilizer is functioning properly. If performed improperly, cleaning and packaging of devices and loading the sterilizer could result in a device that is not sterile, even though the sterilizer is functioning properly.[7]

The prevention of SSI mandates best practices with regard to sterilization of instruments and devices used in surgery. Although it may be difficult to determine exactly why a patient sustains an infection, the risk of infection is increased if an unsterile instrument is used in surgery. Perioperative nurses have a responsibility to ensure that devices used in surgery have been processed according to the most recent guidelines from both the AORN and the AAMI.[5,7]

The best guarantee of a sterile product is proper execution of each step in the sterilization process.[6,7]

SUMMARY

Light can penetrate our perception of black holes. Collaboration among personnel in the CSP, the OR, and the IC helped to identify the causes of failed biologic tests and implement procedures to facilitate safe patient care for those requiring surgery. Respect, understanding, and collaboration are key in addressing patient safety issues.

APPENDIX 1

(Your hospital name)
Report on Positive Test for Sterilizers

Department:_____   Date:_____
Results: Sterilization check positive (failed)
Date positive result was collected:_____   Lot control number:_____
Location of Sterilizer:_____   Room of sterilizer:_____
Date of notification of failure:_____

Type of Sterilization: (check one)
☐ Steam   ☐ Steris(Liquid Peracetic Acid)
☐ Sterrad (II2O2) ☐ Chemical (Other specify)_____
☐ Flash pack

Corrective action taken: (check all appropriate boxes)
☐ Machine taken out of service
☐ Test redone; results "negative"
☐ Test redone; results "positive"
☐ Instruments recalled; no patient involvement
☐ Instruments recalled; patient involvement. Type of action taken. List attached.
☐ PM&C called for service
☐ Inservice/Education (operator)
☐ Vendor repair service called
☐ Other specify_____

Explanation for positive result & machine malfunction: (check all appropriate boxes)
☐   Failure of Validation Test after Repairs
☐   Machine malfunction.
   Specify: ( ) No sterilizers print out for test load.
       ( ) Mechanical Failure caused by Utilities
          (I.e., steam pressure, water shutdown, temperature, etc.).
☐ Improper loading of trays into machine (ETO only)
☐ Improper/Wrong biological indicator used
☐ Incorrect sterilizer settings
☐ Dirty/clogged filters/drain ☐ Operator procedure error
   Specify: ( ) Contaminated spore during transfer procedure
         ( ) Test Expiration date not checked
         ( ) Test did not go through sterilization process
         ( ) Control mislabeled as test
         ( ) Used incorrect settings for testing
         ( ) Auto reader not properly calibrated
Other_____

Additional Information: Patient Involvement ☐ Yes   ☐ No
If yes, identify patient's name and chart number:

MD Notified: [ ] Yes [ ] No MD Name:

Follow-up Actions Necessary:
Contact person:_____   Date:_____Extension:_____

For Department of Infection Control Use Only
Date:_____Reviewed by:_____
Follow-up_____

REFERENCES

1. Amour D, Goulet L, Labadie JF, et al. A model and typology of collaboration between professionals in healthcare organizations. BMC Health Serv Res 2008; 8:188. Available at: http://www.biomedcentral.com/1472-6963/8/188. Accessed February 24, 2010.
2. Larson CE, LaFasto FM. Team work: what must go right/what can go wrong. Newbury Park (CA): Sage Publications; 1989.
3. Joint Commission. Accepted: new and revised hospital elements of performance related to CMS application process. Jt Comm Perspect 2009;29(10):16–9.
4. Association of Operating Room Nurses. Recommended practices for sterilization in the perioperative practice settings. Standards, recommended practices and guidelines. Denver (CO): Association of Operating Room Nurses; 2009.
5. Association for the Advancement of Medical Instrumentation. ANSI/AMMI ST79:2006. Comprehensive guide to steam sterilization and sterility assurance in health care facilities. Arlington (VA): Association for the Advancement of Medical Instrumentation; 2007.
6. Rutala W, Webber D, Healthcare Infection Control Practices Advisory Committee. Guideline for disinfection and sterilization in healthcare facilities, 2008. The Hospital Infection Control Practices Advisory Committee. Available at: http://www.cdc.gov/ncidod/dhqp/pdf/guidelines/Disinfection_Nov_2008.pdf. November 2008.
7. Spry C. Understanding current steam sterilization recommendations and guidelines. AORN J 2008;88(4):537–54.

Strategies for Preventing Sharp Injuries in the Perioperative Setting

Lucille H. Herring, RN, BSN, MS, CIC*

KEYWORDS

- Sharp injuries • Needlesticks • Blood-borne pathogens
- Blood-borne exposure • Perioperative setting

It takes teamwork to eliminate sharp injuries in the perioperative area. There have been strides in the prevention of sharp injuries in the health care setting, with the passage of federal, state, and local legislation and subsequent compliance by health care facilities.[1] However, a recent report revealed that within the perioperative area there has been an increase in exposures to blood and body fluids.[2] The Needlestick Safety and Prevention Act of November 2000 provided stricter guidelines for the protection of health care workers (HCWs), specifically requiring health care employers to provide safety-engineered needles and sharps safety devices whenever they were available in the marketplace.[3] Indeed the revision of the Needlestick Safety and Prevention Act in 2001 specified the use of safer medical devices, annual review of exposure control plans, maintenance of a sharps injury log, and involvement of all team members in evaluating and selecting engineered sharps safety devices.[4] Manufacturers have been and are continuously working with the health care industry to develop safer, clinically effective, and cost-effective devices. Managers and administrators in the perioperative area should comply with this standard and adopt a culture-of-safety attitude regarding exposure to blood and body fluids.

STATISTICS

The US Department of Labor, Occupational Safety and Health Administration (OSHA) estimates that there are approximately 5.6 million health care workers in the United States and that operating room (OR) personnel may have contact with skin or mucous membranes in as many as 50% of operations (range 6.4% to 50.0%). Additionally, needlesticks or cuts may occur in as many as 15% of operations; OR surgeons and first assistants sustain as many as 59.1% of the injuries, with scrub nurses and scrub

Weiler Division, Montefiore Medical Center, Bronx, NY, USA
* 406 Grandview Avenue, Staten Island, NY 10303.
E-mail address: lhhcon@aol.com

Perioperative Nursing Clinics 5 (2010) 501–505
doi:10.1016/j.cpen.2010.10.001
1556-7931/10/$ – see front matter © 2010 Published by Elsevier Inc.

periopnursing.theclinics.com

technicians sustaining the second highest frequency of injuries at 19.1%.[2] Sharp injuries continue to be a challenge in the OR. The more invasive and longer a procedure is, the higher the risk for a sharp injury.[5] The highest-risk procedures are thoracic, trauma, burn, emergency orthopedic, major vascular, intra-abdominal, and gynecologic surgeries. Research indicates that injuries from instruments or sharps devices occur in 7% to 15% of all surgical procedures.[2]

Occupational Safety and Health Administration Standard

A culture of safety must be incorporated into daily work practice. Efforts should be made to eliminate or reduce the use of needles and other sharp-tip instruments. This safety practice is extremely important in the perioperative area. Since the institution of the OSHA Bloodborne Pathogen Standard (29 CRF Part 1910.1030) revised in 2001, most facilities have had an increase in compliance with the sharps safety requirements. This increase is manifested by the acceptance of safety needles and needless intravenous devices. The OSHA blood-borne pathogen document is one of the most important written health care environment mandates that have affected the workplace to prevent the transmission of blood and other potentially infectious materials to health care workers and patients. As a result of the OHSA Bloodborne Pathogen Standard, the health care industry; state health departments; regulatory agencies, including The Joint Commission; and professional organizations, including the American Medical Association, the Association of Perioperative Registered Nurses, the Association for Professionals in Infection Control and Epidemiology, the Society for Healthcare Epidemiology of America, and so forth, have been motivated to change standards of practice and standards of care.[6]

In the surgical setting, there has been a 6.5% increase in sharp injuries, as noted by Jagger and colleagues.[2] Their study showed that from 1993 to 2006, 7186 of the 31,324 total reported sharp injuries were to surgical personnel. After the passage of legislation, there was a decrease in injury rates in nonsurgical settings of 31.6%, but an increased injury rate of 6.5% in surgical settings. A total of 75% of the accidental sticks in the OR occurred when medical devices were in use or passed from one health care worker to another and that the devices associated with the majority of sharps injuries were suture needles (43.4%), scalpel blades (17.0%), and syringes (12.0%).

In the hierarchy of blood-borne pathogen exposure prevention, the first group of strategies calls for administrative policies and procedures to be put into place. A written exposure control plan must be designed to eliminate or minimize employee exposure to blood-borne pathogens. These policies and procedures must also be congruent to real practice and must be monitored. All team members, including surgeons, anesthesiologists, nurses, and technicians, must comply with the OSHA Bloodborne Pathogen Standard, including the written exposure control plan and the local facility infection control guidelines. Appropriate personal protective equipment (PPE) must be provided in adequate amounts by the administration. PPE must be hypoallergenic and be available in a variety of sizes. Doubling gloving, glove liners, and knitted outer gloves also reduce perforations to the innermost glove. The American College of Surgeons recommends the adoption of the double glove and underglove technique to reduce body-fluid exposure caused by glove tears and sharps injuries in surgeons and scrub personnel. In certain delicate operations and in situations where it may compromise the safe conduct of the operation or safety of patients, the surgeon may decide to forgo this safety measure.[7]

Although the perioperative area has always had work practice strategies during surgery, sharps injuries continue to occur. The second group of strategies to prevent sharps injuries in the perioperative area is the implementation of work practice controls. These controls include substituting endoscopic surgery for open surgery when possible and maintaining an attitude and culture of safety when entering the perioperative area.

Before beginning the procedure
1. Organize equipment.
2. Eliminate unnecessary needles and sharps, whenever possible.
3. Control the location of sharps by establishing a *neutral zone*, which is a predetermined space for placing and retrieving sharps. There are hands-free transfer trays and bright-colored (orange) drapes that minimize the risk of sharps injuries and potential contamination.
4. Keep sharps pointed away from the user.

During the surgical procedure
1. Do not hand pass exposed sharps from one person to another.
2. Alert team members when sharps are being passed.
3. Activate the safety feature of devices with engineered sharps-injury prevention features as soon as the procedure is completed.
4. Observe audible (clicks) or visual cues that confirm the feature is locked in place.
5. Maintaining adequate lighting is important.

During cleanup, after the procedure is completed
1. Check procedure trays, waste materials, and linen for exposed sharps before handling.
2. Inspect the container while disposing of sharps.
3. Never put hands in sharps container. Keep hands behind sharps at all times.
4. Be aware that tubing attached to sharps can recoil and lead to injury. Maintain control of both tubing and the device during disposal.
5. After disposing of sharps, visually inspect the sharps container for overfilling and replace containers before they become overfilled.

As a team, on a daily basis
1. Report all injuries or blood/body fluid exposures, sharps injury hazards, and near misses.
2. Include all staff members to participate in surveys and device evaluations.
3. Encourage the team (surgeons, nurses, and technicians) to adhere to safe practices and assist and support coworkers in safer practices.

New work practice strategies for the prevention of sharps injuries, in the perioperative area, must be instituted.

The third group of strategies is engineering controls. Engineering controls are defined as controls that isolate or remove the blood-borne pathogen hazard from the workplace. This strategy group is the area of most innovation. If an effective and clinically appropriate safety-engineered sharp exists, it should be evaluated for possible use. The use of engineering controls (safety devices) does not eliminate the possibility of exposure to blood-borne pathogens. Safety devices alone will not completely eliminate all sharps injuries and bring us to target zero. Surgeons must be encouraged to try clinically appropriate, safety-engineered devices, such as alternative cutting methods (blunt electrocautery and laser devices), when appropriate. In one study, the researchers detected blood splatter from activating retractable phlebotomy and intravascular devices. They showed that there is blood splatter, not obvious to the naked eye, from retracting needles to the mucous membranes of individuals in close proximity. The study also showed the need for HCWs to use PPE while performing phlebotomy and intravenous catheterization.[8] The responsibility is on the HCW to adequately protect themselves against blood splatter from these retractable devices and more improved technology is needed in this area.

The safety mechanism should be integrated into the device. The safety device should keep the workers hands from having to move in front of the sharp. With most safety devices, the user must activate the safety mechanism. The safety device should provide immediate protection after use through disposal. In surgery, technology had to be developed for the specific type of surgery as well as for the instruments and their unique functions. The introduction of any new device must include staff training and follow-up to ensure a positive acceptance of the new safer device.

OSHA, the National Institute for Occupational Safety and Health, the US Centers for Disease Control and Prevention (CDC), and the Department of Health and Human Services published a Safety and Health Information Bulletin regarding the support of the use of blunt-tip suture needles to decrease percutaneous injuries to surgical personnel.[9] Suture needles are the main source of needlesticks in the OR. Sharp-tip suture needles cause 51% to 71% of percutaneous injuries to surgical personnel and are also a risk to patients from possible exposure to the injured staffs' blood. Sharp-tip suture injuries most often occur during suturing of the fascia and muscle. The CDC and other studies have reported the effectiveness of blunt-tip suture needles in decreasing percutaneous injuries.

The American College of Surgeons, in their Statement on Sharps Safety, recommends the adoption of blunt-tip sutures for the closure of fascia and muscle to reduce needlesticks in surgeons and OR personnel.[10] There was some controversy about the effectiveness of using the blunt suture needles in laceration and episiotomy repair during vaginal delivery. One study surveying the issue concluded that in an effort to reduce needlestick injuries, the use of blunt suture needles is safe and effective for repairs at vaginal delivery.[11] Another study concluded that there was no difference in the rate of surgical glove perforation for blunt needles compared with sharp needles used during vaginal laceration repair.[12] Physicians also reported increased difficulty performing the repair with blunt needles. Continuing research is needed on the different types of safety devices and their ease of use and effectiveness.

The issue of blood-borne exposure is a concern in the obstetric area. Although it is an especially serious concern in the delivery room, the issue is also a high priority in the OR when cesarean sections are being performed. Members of the obstetric team have been exposed to umbilical cord blood during the cutting of the cord. One study showed that at least 39% of vaginal deliveries expose at least 1 HCW and 50% of cesarean deliveries expose at least 1 health care worker. A total of 80% of the splashes with body fluids are not reported.[13]

Members of the obstetric team have been exposed to umbilical cord blood during the cutting of the cord. There are several safety devices to prevent exposure to cord blood splatters. These products can safely clamp and cut the cord. There are other devices that safely collect blood samples.

The core component of the strategies for preventing sharps injuries in the perioperative setting involve the implementation and universal compliance with the OSHA Bloodborne Pathogen Standard. The written exposure control plan of the institution must be updated annually or whenever new safety devices and protocols in the perioperative area are implemented. New technology will assist in developing safety devices that meet the needs of health care workers in the perioperative setting. The perioperative team must work with an attitude of safety to prevent sharp injuries.

REFERENCES

1. Herring L. Preventing Hepatitis B transmission in the perioperative environment: focus on policies and procedures. Perioperative Nursing Clinics 2008;3(2): 155–61.
2. Jagger J, Berguer R, Phillips E, et al. Increase in sharps injuries in surgical settings versus nonsurgical setting after passage of national needle stick legislation. J Am Coll Surg 2010;210(4):496–502.
3. Needlestick Safety and Prevention Act of 2000. Pub. L, No. 106-430, 114 Stat. 1901, 2000. Available at: http://frwebgate.access.gpo.gov/cgi-bin/getdoc.cgi?dbname=106_cong_bills&;docid=f:h5178enr.txt.pdf. Accessed June 6, 2010.
4. Department of Labor, Occupational Safety and Health Administration (OSHA). Needlestick Safety and Prevention Act of November 2001, 106th Congress. Public Law 2000;(Pt 1):106–430.
5. White MC, Lynch P. Blood contact and exposures among operating room personnel: a multicenter study. Am J Infect Control 1993;21:243–8.
6. American College of Surgeons, Statement on Sharps Safety, Committee on Perioperative Care. Exposure to blood after use of retractable safety devices. Chicago (IL); 2007.
7. Preventing disease in the operating room. Panel discussion. American College of Surgeons Spring Meeting. Washington, DC, April 29, 1998.
8. Haiduven D, Applegarth S. An experimental method for detecting blood splatter from retractable phlebotomy and intravascular devices. Am J Infect Control 2009; 37(2):127–30.
9. National Institute for Occupational Safety and Health. Use of blunt-tip suture needles to decrease percutaneous injuries to surgical personnel: safety and health information bulletin. Washington, DC: National Institute for Occupational Safety and Health; Publication No. 2008–101.
10. American College of Surgeons. Statement on blunt needles. Bull Am Coll Surg 2005;90:24. Available at: http://www.facs.org/fellows_info/statements/st-52.html. Accessed June 7, 2010.
11. Mornar SJ, Perlow JH. Blunt suture needle use in laceration and episiotomy repair at vaginal delivery. Am J Obstet Gynecol 2008;198(5):e14–5.
12. Wilson LK, Sullivan S, Goodnight W. The use of blunt needles does not reduce glove perforation during obstetrical laceration repair. Am J Obstet Gynecol 2008;199(6):641.
13. Stoker R. Cutting the cord. Managing Infection Control 2006;(Pt 2):34–47. Available at: http://www.manageinfection.com. Accessed October 18, 2010.

Index

Note: Page numbers of article titles are in **boldface** type.

A

AAMI. See *Association for the Advancement of Medical Instrumentation (AAMI) standards.*
Anesthesia/anesthetics
    as risk for health care–acquired infections, **427–441**
        catheter-associated infection, 430–431
        described, 427–428
        equipment-related infection, 435–437
        infusate-associated infection, 430–431
        interruption of skin barrier via devices that enter intravascular system and, 430
        interruption of skin barrier via devices that penetrate spinal column and, 428–430
        intubation-related infection, 435–437
        mechanical ventilation–related infection, 435–437
        prevention of
            anesthesia team in, 437–438
            in anesthesia personnel, 438–439
    equipment for, infections related to, 435–437
    personnel administering, health care–acquired infections in, prevention of, 438–439
Antisepsis
    skin
        described, 457–458
        surgical, **457–477.** See also *Skin antisepsis, surgical.*
        surgical hand, **443–448.** See also *Surgical hand antisepsis (SHA).*
Antiseptic agents, in skin antisepsis
    activity of, 462
    studies of, 464–465
Association for the Advancement of Medical Instrumentation (AAMI) standards, in flash
    sterilization of operating room, 494–495

B

Biologic cultures, positive, found during flash sterilization of operating room, **489–500.**
    See also *Operating room, flash sterilization of, increased positive biologic cultures
    found during.*
Black holes, described, 489

C

Catheter(s), infections related to, 430–431
    prevention of, 431–434
    UTI, **449–456.** See also *Catheter-associated urinary tract infection (CAUTI).*
Catheter-associated urinary tract infection (CAUTI), **449–456**
    causes of, 450–451
    described, 449–450

Perioperative Nursing Clinics 5 (2010) 507–510
doi:10.1016/S1556-7931(10)00092-6
1556-7931/10/$ – see front matter © 2010 Elsevier Inc. All rights reserved.

United States Postal Service

Statement of Ownership, Management, and Circulation
(All Periodicals Publications Except Requestor Publications)

1. Publication Title	2. Publication Number	3. Filing Date
Perioperative Nursing Clinics	0 2 4 - 5 3 5	9/15/1)

4. Issue Frequency	5. Number of Issues Published Annually	6. Annual Subscription Price
Mar, Jun, Sep, Dec	4	$116.00

7. Complete Mailing Address of Known Office of Publication (Not printer) (Street, city, county, state, and ZIP+4®)

Elsevier Inc.
360 Park Avenue South
New York, NY 10010-1710

Contact Person
Stephen Bushing
Telephone (Include area code)
215-239-3688

8. Complete Mailing Address of Headquarters or General Business Office of Publisher (Not printer)

Elsevier Inc., 360 Park Avenue South, New York, NY 10010-1710

9. Full Names and Complete Mailing Addresses of Publisher, Editor, and Managing Editor (Do not leave blank)

Publisher (Name and complete mailing address)

Kim Murphy, Elsevier, Inc., 1600 John F. Kennedy Blvd. Suite 1800, Philadelphia, PA 19103-2899

Editor (Name and complete mailing address)

Katie Hartner, Elsevier, Inc., 1600 John F. Kennedy Blvd. Suite 1800, Philadelphia, PA 19103-2899

Managing Editor (Name and complete mailing address)

Catherine Bewick, Elsevier, Inc., 1600 John F. Kennedy Blvd. Suite 1800, Philadelphia, PA 19103-2899

10. Owner (Do not leave blank. If the publication is owned by a corporation, give the name and address of the corporation immediately followed by the names and addresses of all stockholders owning or holding 1 percent or more of the total amount of stock. If not owned by a corporation, give the names and addresses of the individual owners. If owned by a partnership or other unincorporated firm, give its name and address as well as those of each individual owner. If the publication is published by a nonprofit organization, give its name and address.)

Full Name	Complete Mailing Address
Wholly owned subsidiary of	4520 East-West Highway
Reed/Elsevier, US holdings	Bethesda, MD 20814

11. Known Bondholders, Mortgagees, and Other Security Holders Owning or Holding 1 Percent or More of Total Amount of Bonds, Mortgages, or Other Securities. If none, check box   ☐ None

Full Name	Complete Mailing Address
N/A	

12. Tax Status (For completion by nonprofit organizations authorized to mail at nonprofit rates) (Check one)
The purpose, function, and nonprofit status of this organization and the exempt status for federal income tax purposes:
☐ Has Not Changed During Preceding 12 Months
☐ Has Changed During Preceding 12 Months (Publisher must submit explanation of change with this statement)

PS Form 3526, September 2007 (Page 1 of 3 (Instructions Page 3)) PSN 7530-01-000-9931 PRIVACY NOTICE: See our Privacy policy in www.usps.com

---

13. Publication Title	14. Issue Date for Circulation Data Below
Perioperative Nursing Clinics	September 2010

15. Extent and Nature of Circulation		Average No. Copies Each Issue During Preceding 12 Months	No. Copies of Single Issue Published Nearest to Filing Date
a. Total Number of Copies (Net press run)		583	527
b. Paid Circulation (By Mail and Outside the Mail)	(1) Mailed Outside-County Paid Subscriptions Stated on PS Form 3541 (Include paid distribution above nominal rate, advertiser's proof copies, and exchange copies)	292	280
	(2) Mailed In-County Paid Subscriptions Stated on PS Form 3541 (Include paid distribution above nominal rate, advertiser's proof copies, and exchange copies)		
	(3) Paid Distribution Outside the Mails Including Sales Through Dealers and Carriers, Street Vendors, Counter Sales, and Other Paid Distribution Outside USPS®	7	9
	(4) Paid Distribution by Other Classes Mailed Through the USPS (e.g. First-Class Mail®)		
c. Total Paid Distribution (Sum of 15b (1), (2), (3), and (4))	▶	299	289
d. Free or Nominal Rate Distribution (By Mail and Outside the Mail)	(1) Free or Nominal Rate Outside-County Copies Included on PS Form 3541	59	47
	(2) Free or Nominal Rate In-County Copies Included on PS Form 3541		
	(3) Free or Nominal Rate Copies Mailed at Other Classes Through the USPS (e.g. First-Class Mail)		
	(4) Free or Nominal Rate Distribution Outside the Mail (Carriers or other means)		
e. Total Free or Nominal Rate Distribution (Sum of 15d (1), (2), (3) and (4)	▶	59	47
f. Total Distribution (Sum of 15c and 15e)	▶	358	336
g. Copies not Distributed (See instructions to publishers #4 (page #3))	▶	225	191
h. Total (Sum of 15f and g)	▶	583	527
i. Percent Paid (15c divided by 15f times 100)		83.52%	86.01%

16. Publication of Statement of Ownership

If the publication is a general publication, publication of this statement is required. Will be printed in the December 2010 issue of this publication.   Publication not required

17. Signature and Title of Editor, Publisher, Business Manager, or Owner   Date

Stephen R. Bushing – Fulfillment/Inventory Specialist   September 15, 2010

Stephen R. Bushing – Fulfillment/Inventory Specialist

I certify that all information furnished on this form is true and complete. I understand that anyone who furnishes false or misleading information on this form or who omits material or information requested on the form may be subject to criminal sanctions (including fines and imprisonment) and/or civil sanctions (including civil penalties).

PS Form 3526, September 2007 (Page 2 of 3)

Moving?

Make sure your subscription moves with you!

To notify us of your new address, find your **Clinics Account Number** (located on your mailing label above your name), and contact customer service at:

Email: **journalscustomerservice-usa@elsevier.com**

800-654-2452 (subscribers in the U.S. & Canada)
314-447-8871 (subscribers outside of the U.S. & Canada)

Fax number: 314-447-8029

Elsevier Health Sciences Division
Subscription Customer Service
3251 Riverport Lane
Maryland Heights, MO 63043

*To ensure uninterrupted delivery of your subscription, please notify us at least 4 weeks in advance of move.